Managing & Leading

44 Lessons Learned for Pharmacists

Paul W. Bush and Stuart G. Walesh

American Society of Health–System Pharmacists®
Bethesda, Maryland

Managing and Leading: 44 Lessons Learned for Pharmacists is based on the work, *Managing and Leading: 52 Lessons Learned for Engineers,* Copyright 2004, American Society of Civil Engineers. (http://pubs.asce.org)

Any correspondence regarding this publication should be sent to the publisher, American Society of Health-System Pharmacists, 7272 Wisconsin Avenue, Bethesda, MD 20814, attention: Special Publishing.

The information presented herein reflects the opinions of the contributors and advisors. It should not be interpreted as an official policy of ASHP or as an endorsement of any product.

Director, Special Publishing: Jack Bruggeman

Acquisitions Editor: Jack Bruggeman

Senior Editorial Project Manager: Dana Battaglia

Editorial Resources Manager: Bill Fogle

Page and cover design: Carol Barrer

Page layout: David Wade

Library of Congress Cataloging-in-Publication Data

Bush, Paul W.
  Managing and leading : 44 lessons learned for pharmacists / Paul W. Bush and Stuart G. Walesh.
     p. cm.
  "Managing and Leading: 44 Lessons Learned for Pharmacists is based on the work, Managing and Leading: 52 Lessons Learned for Engineers, Copyright 2004, American Society of Civil Engineers."
  ISBN 978-1-58528-170-1
  1. Pharmacy management. I. Walesh, S. G. II. Walesh, S. G. Managing and leading. III. Title.

RS100.B87 2008
615'.1068—dc22
                        2008005252

ISBN 978-1-58528-170-1

Acknowledgments

Jack Bruggeman, ASHP Acquisitions and Special Publishing Director, created the opportunity to write this book when he recognized that managing and leading pharmacists was similar to managing and leading engineers. With the assistance of the health system pharmacy residents at the Medical University of South Carolina, Dr. Stuart G. Walesh's book, *Managing and Leading: 52 Lessons Learned for Engineers,* was rewritten to be applicable to pharmacists.

Drs. Heather Kokko, Kuldip Patel, Christopher Fortier, Jennifer Jastrzembski, Matthew Maughan, and Carolyn Smith revised lessons, adding new content and references to weave the pharmacy perspective throughout the book. They drew ideas and examples from many past and current pharmacy leaders, including several Harvey A. K. Whitney Award recipients.

Co-author Paul Bush notes that his wife, Julie, provided guidance, critiques of ideas, and support throughout the project. Co-author Stu Walesh acknowledges the cooperation of ASCE Press and recalls the authors, former students, seminar and workshop participants, clients, colleagues, and friends who contributed to the original managing and leading book.

About the Authors

Dr. Paul W. Bush, Pharm.D., M.B.A., FASHP has more than 30 years of experience as a clinically oriented pharmacy leader. He earned a B.S. in Pharmacy from the University of Michigan, and a Pharm.D. and M.B.A. from Wayne State University.

Bush has held positions as clinical pharmacist, multi-hospital system clinical director, corporate pharmacy director, academic medical center pharmacy director, associate professor, director of graduate pharmacy education, director of dual degree Pharm.D./M.B.A. program and residency program director. He has been actively involved in residency training since 1992 and has served as a member of the ASHP Commission on Credentialing. He has established and directed technician training programs in both Michigan and South Carolina.

He has authored and co-authored chapters in several publications including *Handbook of Institutional Pharmacy Practice, Financial Management Basics for Health System Pharmacists,* and *Pharmacy Certified Technician Training Manual,* and numerous articles and presentations.

Bush is a member of ASHP, ACCP, and APhA. He has served as member, board member, chair, and president of state and national committees and organizations. In 1999, he received the Distinguished Alumni Award from Wayne State University; in 2001, he was elected Fellow of the American Society of Health-System Pharmacists; and in 2005 he received the South Carolina League of Nursing Award for Excellence.

Dr. Stuart G. Walesh, Ph.D., P.E., Hon.M.ASCE, has over 40 years of engineering, education, and management-leadership experience in the government and private sectors. He earned a B.S. in Civil Engineering at Valparaiso University, an M.S.E. at The Johns Hopkins University, and a Ph.D. from the University of Wisconsin-Madison. He has functioned as a project manager, department head, discipline manager, marketer, professor, dean of an engineering college, and independent consultant.

As an independent consultant, Dr. Walesh provides managing, leading, engineering, education/training, and marketing services. Clients include professional service firms, government agencies, and professional societies. Managing and leading are of special interest including the extent to which basic managing and leading principles apply to various disciplines. Accordingly, Walesh was pleased to have the opportunity to co-author this book for the use in the pharmacy profession.

Walesh authored *Urban Surface Water Management* (Wiley, 1989), *Engineering Your Future* (ASCE Press, 2000), *Flying Solo: How to Start an Individual Practitioner Consulting Business* (Hannah Publishing, 2000), and *Managing and Leading: 52 Lessons Learned for Engineers* (ASCE Press, 2004). Walesh is author or co-author of over 200 publications and presentations and has facilitated or presented hundreds of workshops, seminars, webinars, and meetings throughout the U.S.

Walesh is a member of and has chaired state and national committees and groups within various professional organizations. In 1995, he received the Public Service Award from the Consulting Engineers of Indiana; in 1998, the Distinguished Service Citation from the College of Engineering at the University of Wisconsin; in 2003, the Excellence in Civil Engineering Education Leadership Award presented by American Society of Civil Engineers (ASCE); in 2004, he was elected an Honorary Member of ASCE; in 2005, he was elected a Diplomate of the American Academy of Water Resource Engineers; in 2007, he was named Engineer of the Year by the Indiana Society of Professional Engineers and received a Distinguished Service Award from the National Society of Professional Engineers.

Foreword

I find this publication a significant and unique addition to the pharmacy literature which should be considered not only by current leaders but by all pharmacists, PGY1 residency directors, and Colleges of Pharmacy students and faculty. I am pleased that it is a concise and practical handbook that I recommend be on every current and aspiring pharmacy leader and manager's desk. Paul Bush has brought to this publication his 30 years of experience in pharmacy leadership and involved his current and past administrative residents to bring it a view from the "younger generation of leaders and mangers." They should be commended for their efforts.

Pharmacy leadership and management has never been as demanding, multifaceted, complex and critical as it is today and hence the need for this information. Current formal "Big L" leaders (Director, Associate, Assistant, Coordinator, Supervisor, Lead, etc.) and managers must daily juggle:

- Working effectively with people, both their staff and others throughout the organization
- Being financially responsible for a major part of the organization's expense and revenue budget, most of which they and their staff don't directly control, i.e., write medication orders
- Making sure all the ever changing regulatory and legal "bases" are covered for medications which are everywhere in the organization, not just in the pharmacy
- Ensuring that medications do not harm patients everywhere they are used
- Develop and maintain good working relationships not only with the medical and nursing staff but with administration, finance, and virtually every other organizational department
- Lead the organizational efforts to improve the medication use system for all the patients, from procuring, prescribing, dispensing, monitoring through medication administration and appropriate charging
- Anticipate and innovate to ensure patients benefit from the new developments in health care
- Keep up not only with the barrage of information such as e-mails, voice mails, journals, newsletters, push news, list serves, but their own self-development
- And other duties as assigned

While these varied responsibilities may seem daunting, they also require a highly scientifically educated and trained person to be able to switch into the art of leading and managing where there are very few true principles as there are in science. Many current and aspiring pharmacy leaders and managers have not benefited from formal training in the art of leading and managing pharmacies. Likewise these skills are not just needed by the formal "Big L" leaders, but every pharmacist as a "Little L" leader on their shift or in their practice needs to employ the leadership techniques found in this book to ensure their maximum impact.

Effective pharmacist leadership, both "Big L and Little L," is crucial to the continuing evolution of pharmacy services. Having separated from early medical practitioners as the unique knowledge of specific medications developed, past pharmacy leaders saw the need for pharmacists to apply their drug knowledge to help patients minimize diseases. In health-systems this evolution included compounding intravenous admixtures, developing unit dose drug distribution systems, handling investigational drugs, utilizing formulary systems to promote rational cost effective prescribing, compounding radiopharmaceuticals, moving out of the pharmacy to practice in the patient care areas along side physicians and nurses, computerizing systems, integrating automation, and championing patient medication safety. Only pharmacist leaders can continue this evolution into the future because they understand where the unmet needs are. My leadership published research (*AJHP* 2005) has shown that over the next decade 80% of the current health-system directors of pharmacy and 77% of the middle managers anticipate retiring. These data also indicate that there may not be enough interest by current practitioners to fill these vacancies with pharmacists. The most often cited reason for not being interested in leadership positions is too many competing responsibilities and having to give up their clinical practice. If there are not enough pharmacists to take on these vacant leadership positions then non-pharmacists will have to be utilized which may not be in the best interest of patients and pharmacy staffs.

This book as a primer and handbook can assist leaders, managers and all pharmacists to be more effective. It is filled with non-pharmacy quotes that offer a philosophical backdrop to each topic or lesson. The 44 lessons are conveniently organized into eight parts; personal roles, goals and development, communication, learning and teaching, improving personal and organizational productivity, meetings, marketing, building mutually beneficial employee-employer partnerships and the broad view. Each lesson very effectively contains pharmacy examples, suggestions for application and using the material, related lessons, sources cited in the lesson for further study, suggested supplemental sources, e-newsletters, and applicable websites. The use of key concepts tables make it easy to use as a just-in-time resource.

There are the typical topics you would expect, such as, how to set goals, using questions in communication, establishing culture, the difference between leadership and management, etc but there are many unique topics that add dimensions not usually found in such publications. The following are a few examples.

- Too much of a good thing. Avoiding the pitfalls of too much experience.
- Courage: real and counterfeit. Rising change and confronting the unknown.

- Afraid of dying, or not having lived? Realizing our dreams instead of living with regret.
- Balance high tech and high touch. Mixing technology with human contact.

Readers will benefit from the variety of "pearls" that will enable them to be more efficient and effective no matter what their job responsibilities.

Sara J. White, M.S., FASHP
Director of Pharmacy (retired)
Pharmacy Leadership Coach
Mountain View, California
January 2008

Preface

Managing and Leading: 44 Lessons Learned for Pharmacists is designed to help health system pharmacists manage and lead primarily in their practice but also in their community and other activities.

The 44 lessons in this book present useful ideas for ways to more effectively work with staff or colleagues. Many of the lessons include content that is directly related to memorable and sometimes challenging situations that we have experienced during our careers. Each lesson contains an essay that offers at least one idea or principle for honing management and leadership effectiveness. Following each lesson are pragmatic suggestions for ways to apply the ideas using application tools and techniques such as action items, guidelines, do's and don'ts, checklists, forms, and resource materials including articles, papers, books, e-newsletters, and websites. The goal is to enable you to practice even better stewardship with who you are and what and who you know.

Many approaches to use of this book are possible, the most obvious of which is to consecutively read all 44 lessons on one or more sittings. A more focused approach is to select a lesson or group of lessons from the Contents or Index that resonates with your current need. A third option is to select one lesson each week and work through the lessons over 11 or 12 months.

Upon reading a lesson, you may determine its message has potential value for you. If so, commit to putting the underlying ideas or principles into practice, at least on a trial basis, and experiment with some of the suggestions. Perhaps you will leverage the lessons into a new life-long management and leadership habit. Even if you don't change your method of working, you will have examined and confirmed it on its merits.

Counseling, teaching, training, and mentoring are other possible uses of *Managing and Leading*. The lessons in the book can be utilized for staff aspiring to gain managing and leading positions or to improve their supervisory skills. This could be facilitated by establishing a weekly or monthly "leadership forum" focusing on one lesson during each session.

The book can also be used by preceptors for student health system pharmacy management experiential rotations or postgraduate year one residency training. Individual students or residents could be asked to review selected lessons and offer their views in an administrative rounds or journal club setting. *Managing and Leading* could also be used as a supplemental text for pharmacy management courses. Finally, mentors might assign their protégés one or more related lessons for self-study and discussion.

Managing and Leading: 44 Lessons Learned for Pharmacists is intended to support current leaders and encourage pharmacists, residents and students to pursue management and leadership roles within and outside of their profession.

Paul W. Bush, Pharm.D., M.B.A., FASHP
Stuart G. Walesh, Ph.D., P.E., Hon.M.ASCE

Contents

Part 1: Personal Roles, Goals, and Development

Lessons

Part 2: Communication

Lessons

Part 3: Learning and Teaching

Lessons

Part 4: Improving Personal and Organizational Productivity

Lessons

Part 5: Meetings

Lessons

Part 6: Marketing

Lessons

Part 7: Building Mutually Beneficial Employee-Employer Partnerships

Lessons

Part 8: The Broad View

Lessons

Part 1

||||||||||||||||||||||||||||||||||||||||||||||||||||||||||||||||||||||||||||||||

Personal Roles, Goals, and Development

"Get your ducks in a row" has always been one of my favorite expressions. Another is "begin with the end in mind." These expressions emphasize the importance of preparation and, while they apply to groups and individuals, the latter is relevant here.

If we aspire to manage and lead individuals, projects, organizations, and change, we must first get our personal "ducks in a row." This requires selecting roles, setting goals and acquiring and developing supportive knowledge, skills and attitudes that have proven to be effective. Helping you get your personal act together by thinking about and embracing that knowledge-skills-attitudes set is the purpose of the 11 lessons in this section.

Lesson 1

Leading, Managing, and Producing

|||||||||||||||||||||||||||||||||||||||||||||||||||||||||||||||||||||||||||||||||||||||||||||||||

Leaders are people who do the right things;
managers are people who do things right.
Both roles are crucial,
but they differ profoundly.

— Warren G. Bennis

One model for organizations, such as healthcare systems, academic departments, or colleges of pharmacy, is that wholeness, vitality, and resiliency require attention to three different, but inextricably related, on-going functions: leading, managing, and producing. Another way of looking at leading, managing, and producing is to think of them as the three D's: deciding, directing, and doing.

The three different, but complementary, efforts essential to an organization's success, may be further explained as follows:

- Leading involves deciding what ought to be done or determining where an organization should go. When we are in a leading or deciding mode, helpful knowledge and skills include visioning, communication, honesty and integrity, goal setting and related strategizing, continuous learning, courage, calmness in crises, tolerance for ambiguity, and creativity.

Leadership works through people and culture.
It's soft and hot.
Management works through hierarchy and systems.
It's harder and cooler.

— John P. Kotter

- Managing focuses on directing who is doing what when. When we are in a managing or directing mode, useful knowledge and skills include communication, delegation of authority, planning, resource acquisition and allocation, and monitoring.
- Producing involves doing what has been decided as a result of leading and what is being directed via managing. When we are in a producing or doing mode, helpful knowledge and skills include clinical and technical competence, focus, persistence, and teamwork.

The metaphor of a three-legged stool suggests how attention to leading, managing, and producing creates a stable organization—one that cannot easily be "knocked over." While an organization or group might temporarily survive balanced on two of the three legs, all three legs are needed for long-term survival. For example, a leaderless pharmacy department might do well for several years by balancing on two legs such as excellent management and service capabilities, but eventually be toppled because it lacked the third leg. That leg is leadership, especially the ability to see and act on changes in client and customer needs and the means to serve those needs. Leadership author Warren G. Bennis[1] says:

> Many an institution is very well-managed and very poorly led. It may excel in the ability to handle each day all the routine inputs, yet may never ask whether the routine should be done at all.

Consider another example of the need for three strong legs, with each carrying its share of the weight. Picture a pharmacy consulting firm led by a visionary and staffed with individuals willing to produce, but lacking the managing leg, that is, effective project managers. This firm is likely to fail because it lacks the ability to translate the vision to profitable services and deliverables.

Assuming you agree that each organization or group striving to be successful has leading (deciding), managing (directing), and producing (doing) responsibilities, consider the manner in which these corporate responsibilities might be met. More specifically; consider the matter of individual responsibility in achieving the three organizational responsibilities.

In what might be called the traditional segregated model, the three functions reside in three separate groups of personnel. The vast majority of employees or group members are the doers or producers, a distinctly different and much smaller group of managers are the directors, and one person, or perhaps a very small group, leads.

Another traditional way of viewing the production, management, and leadership functions is the linear model. An aspiring and successful individual begins in a production mode and then passes linearly through management and into leadership. Rather than being a trait that many can possess, albeit to different degrees, leadership is considered the end of the line or ultimate destination for a very few. But is this the optimum way for the modern or future organization or group to meet its leading, managing, and producing responsibilities? Probably not.

An organization will be stronger if what used to be the three organizational responsibilities now also become individual responsibilities. The goal should be to enable each member of the organization or group to be a decider, a director, and a doer. While the relative "amounts" of leading, managing, and producing will vary markedly among individuals in the organization or group, everyone should be expected and enabled to do all three in accordance with their individual characteristics.

If you want to build a ship,
don't drum up the people to gather wood,
divide up the work and give orders.
Instead, teach them to yearn for the vast and endless sea.

— Antoine de Saint-Exupery

This shared responsibility organizational model, in contrast with the traditional segregated model, is much more likely to tap, draw on, and benefit from the diverse aspirations, talents, and skills that should be present within the organization or group. Because essentially all members are fully involved, the shared responsibility entity is in a much better position to synergistically build on internal strengths, to cooperatively diminish internal weaknesses, and to learn about and be prepared to respond to external threats and opportunities.

In conclusion, leading, managing, and doing are not defined only or even primarily by position. Instead, the principal determinate is individual knowledge, skills, and attitudes. Anyone at any level within an organization or group, can and should, exercise deciding, directing, and doing as needs and opportunities arise.

Suggestions for Applying Ideas

Review examples of the distinctions between leading, managing, and producing (or deciding, directing, and doing) such as the following:

TABLE 1-1. DISTINCTION BETWEEN LEADING, MANAGING, AND PRODUCING		
LEADING	**MANAGING**	**PRODUCING**
Deciding what ought to be done	Directing how things will be done, who will do them and when	Doing what we know has to be done or what we are asked to do
What do we want to accomplish?	How can we best accomplish it	Do it
Determine if the ladder is leaning against the right wall[4]	Determine how to efficiently climb the ladder[4]	Climb the ladder and go over the wall[4]
Select jungle to conquer[4]	Sharpen machetes, write policy and procedure manuals, establish working schedules[4]	Cut through the jungle[4]

Look for and act on leadership events.

▢ Health system pharmacy is a rapidly changing, highly regulated, and competitive environment, where a need exists for pharmacists to seek "leadership events" at all levels of the department.[2] A leadership event is defined as "some situation in organizational life, which contains for an individual, an unfilled need for leadership."[3]

▢ Examples of possible leadership events are a failing medication management process, a need to develop a new service in an outpatient clinic, a need to comply with accreditation standards, an increasingly irrelevant curriculum in a college department, and organizing a new type of employee gathering within an organization.

▢ The ability of a person to choose her or his view on a project or task is an important concept as it opens to the potential leader the possibility of changing other participants' views of the task. The point: There are many ways to look at situations ranging from, at one end of the spectrum, mundane, routine and more of the same to, at the other end of the spectrum, a unique opportunity for improvement and achievement. To take possession of a leadership event implies that there will be change. Seek out opportunities for leadership events, embrace them with optimism and hope.[2]

Having identified a potential leadership event, move, as appropriate, through the following process:

▢ Confirm that your leadership is required and feasible. (Have a purpose).

▢ Begin with the end in mind.[4]

▢ Determine the stakeholders.

▢ Estimate what "costs" and "benefits" might be incurred, or perceived to be incurred, by each stakeholder.

▢ Have a vision. Engage others to share your event meaning and endorse your leadership.

▢ Sustain the network of stakeholders by communicating and reinforcing roles.

- Organize the stakeholders to achieve common goals.
- Recognize when goals have been achieved, and celebrate!
- Experience strongly indicates that each of us is surrounded by leadership opportunities, regardless of our formal position.

Nothing is orderly until man takes hold of it.
Everything in creation lies around loose.

— Henry Ward Beecher

Think about the do's and don'ts of effective managing[5]

- Managers should be leaders. Remember "Managers do right things, and leaders do things right."
- Stay in touch – communicate with all employees at all levels.
- Listen, consider, act, provide feedback, and give credit to those who deserve it.
- Plan – have a mission and vision. Focus on an agreed upon plan to achieve the mission and vision.
- Put yourself "in their shoes." Have sensitivity and appropriate timing when addressing problems, issues, or change events.
- Continually guide and encourage the staff toward achieving goals within limits of the abilities and resources available.
- Emphasize quality—"we do it right the first time, every time."
- Reward competence.
- Create and follow standards of practice and supervision in cooperation with those people affected by the standards.
- Maintain a good work climate comprised of respect, trust, and a sense of pride.
- Protect your workers from the bureaucracy to instill a sense of security.
- Build a team where everyone know their jobs but buys into mutual goals and works together to accomplish those goals.

~~~~~~~~~~~~~~~~~~~~~~

Manage from the left (brain);
lead from the right.

— Stephen R. Covey

Evaluate your managing and leading potential by comparing your personal profile to that of the highly accomplished pharmacist, Harvey A. K. Whitney

⊡ Whitney's achievements included occupying the position of Chief Pharmacist at the University Hospital in Ann Arbor Michigan for 20 years, establishing the first pharmacy internship program (now known as a pharmacy residency program), developing a small subset of American Pharmacists Association members interested in hospital pharmacy and creating and presiding over American Society of Hospital Pharmacy as well as creating the *American Journal of Hospital Pharmacy.*

⊡ The following are attributes needed by all leaders[2]:

- Competence
- Knowledge
- Trustworthiness
- Being an effective listener
- Respecting others
- Compassion
- Observing fairness
- Generosity
- Openness

⊡ The following practices have also been associated with effective leadership[2]:

- Taking risks—drives change
- Inspire excellence and provide clarity through a vision
- Build and empower teams

- Foster development of talents
- Communicate effectively
- Listen and keep informed
- Develop relationships
- Lead by example
- Celebrate success

How do you stack up? Using Harvey A. K. Whitney as a benchmark, what are your managing and leading strengths and weaknesses?

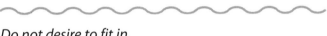

Do not desire to fit in.
Desire to lead.

— Gwendolyn Brooks

Study one or more of the following sources cited in this lesson

1. Bennis WG. *Why Leaders Can't Lead—The Unconscious Conspiracy Continues.* San Francisco: Jossey-Bass Publishers; 1989:17.
2. Wollenberg KG, Bush PW. Leadership. In: Brown TR, ed. *Handbook of Institutional Pharmacy Practice.* Bethesda, MD: American Society of Health-System Pharmacists; 2006:217–227.
3. Parkin J. Choosing to lead. *J Manage Eng.* 1997;(Jan./Feb.):62–63.
4. Covey SR. *The 7 Habits of Highly Effective People.* New York: Simon & Schuster; 1990.
5. Brown TR, ed. *Handbook of Institutional Pharmacy Practice.* Bethesda, MD: American Society of Health-System Pharmacists; 2006:125–132.

Study one or more of the following supplemental sources

- DePue M. *Leadership is An Art.* New York: Dell Publishing Company, 1989.

- Gerber R. *Leadership the Eleanor Roosevelt Way: Timeless Strategies from the First Lady of Courage.* Upper Saddle River, NJ: Prentice Hall Press, 2002.

- Hunter JC. *The Servant: A Simple Story About the True Essence of Leadership.* Rocklin, CA; Prima Publishing, 1998.

- Kotter JP. *John Kotter on What Leaders Really Do.* Cambridge, MA: Harvard Business Review, 1999.

- Maxwell JC. *The 21 Irrefutable Laws of Leadership.* Nashville, TN: Thomas Nelson Publishers, 1998.

- Peterson AM. Chapter 5: Leadership. In: Peterson AM, ed. *Managing Pharmacy Practice: Principles, Strategies, and Systems.* Washington, DC: CRC Press; 2004:57–66.

- Peterson AM. Managing professionals. In: Peterson AM, ed. *Managing Pharmacy Practice: Principles, Strategies, and Systems.* Washington, DC: CRC Press; 2004:57–66.

You young lieutenants have to realize that
your platoon is like a piece of spaghetti.
You cannot push it.
You have to get out front and pull it.

— George S. Patton, Jr.

Subscribe to one or more of these e-newsletters

- "Leading Effectively e-Newsletter," a free monthly newsletter from the Center for Creative Leadership. Provides "tools, tips, and advice to practicing managers who face the daily challenges of leading." Includes short articles and presents case studies and results of polls. Offers programs, products, and publications. To subscribe go to http://www.ccl.org.

- "Leadership Wired" is a free semi-monthly newsletter from John C. Maxwell. Typically included are short articles, book reviews, and quotes. To subscribe, go to http://www.injoy.com.

Visit one or more of these websites

■ "American Management Association" (http://www.amanet.org) is provided by the AMA, which was founded in 1923 and is "dedicated to building the knowledge, skills, and behaviors that will help business professionals and their organizations grow and prosper." Leads users to education and training opportunities including seminars, conferences, forums, books, research, and self-study courses. Includes many previously presented short, application-oriented, articles.

■ "Academy of Management" (http://www.aomonline.org/) is maintained by the AOM. Established in 1936, the AOM is "a leading professional association for scholars dedicated to creating and disseminating knowledge about management and organizations." Includes meeting announcements, products and services, and a means for retrieval of articles previously published in the Academy's journals.

■ "Center for Creative Leadership" (http://www.ccl.org) is maintained by the Center for Creative Leadership where the mission is "to advance the understanding, practice and development of leadership for the benefit of society worldwide." Describes the Center's leadership program, products, and leadership conferences and explains the function of various special groups.

A leader is a dealer in hope.

— Napoleon Bonapart

Lesson 2

Roles, Then Goals
||||||||||||||||||||||||||||||||||||||||||||||||||||||||||||||||||||||||||||||||||||||

One man cannot do right in one department of life
whilst he is occupied doing wrong in other departments.
Life is one indivisible whole.

— Mahatma Gandhi

In the first part of the new year, many of us make—and often break – annual resolutions or goals. Our good intentions don't pan out. Goals deemed worthy on January 1 no longer seem to warrant special efforts. What's wrong?

One answer may be that while our resolutions and goals are well-intentioned, they lack context or perspective. Our frustrating failure frequently follows from lack of relevance of the resolutions and goals to our overall life. Our resolutions and goals may be too narrowly focused, most likely on our job, to the exclusion of our other areas of responsibility and opportunity. As a result, our goals are out of "sync" with our total being— our true range of abilities, interests, and aspirations. Perhaps our goals are solely or overly job focused because we think it's the pragmatic or responsible thing to do. After all, we "must be practical," especially as clinically minded can-do professionals!

One way to enhance the relevance of our goals is to cast them in terms of our desired roles. Adopt a holistic approach. That is, we should first select our key roles in life, at least for the foreseeable future. Then make resolutions or establish goals that will help us fulfill those valued roles. This roles first-goals second idea comes from the Covey Leadership Center. Speaker and author Stephen Covey explained it this way[2]:

> One of the major problems that arises when people work to become more effective in life is that they don't think broadly enough. They lose the sense of proportion, the balance, the natural ecology necessary to effective living. They may get consumed by work.

An example of a non-work role that is likely to be shared by many clinical professionals is parent. Other common non-work roles are daughter, son, wife, husband, grandparent, neighbor, athlete, friend, member of a religious group, and community leader. As used in the preceding sentence, "common" means a role likely to be held by many individuals, as opposed to a rare role. "Common" does not mean unimportant.

Examples of work-related roles likely to be held by pharmacists and other healthcare professionals are preceptor, educator, clinical practitioner, administrator, project manager, mentor, committee member, and officer in a professional, business, or service organization. Frankly, today's typical healthcare professional probably has more work-related roles than his or her counterpart did a decade or so ago. Such added expectations are one manifestation of the changing world of work. All the more reason for each of us to perform a role check.

Although many of us share some roles, our interpretations of success in any given role will vary widely. Consider, for example, the non-work role of a community member. Some of us probably think that we successfully fulfill our community responsibilities by quietly going about our business. Others would say that success in the community role requires proactive involvement in our immediate neighborhood or perhaps an even higher profile leadership role in the community at large. All are legitimate, especially if they are done by design.

Purpose is what gives life meaning.

— Charles Henry Parkhurst

Clearly, we can establish goals without first defining roles. The danger is that we will inadvertently omit or diminish important segments of our being. We risk incurring deep regrets that cannot be remedied. In contrast, the suggested "roles—then goals" process has the advantage of causing each of us to strive for balance in our life. Thomas L. Brown, management writer and speaker, said it this way: "…you cannot balance your personal and professional life unless there is substantial weight on both ends.[2]"

Suggestions for Applying Ideas

Experiment with the roles first goals second idea advocated in this lesson by at least starting the process. Create and fill out a table like the following:

TABLE 2-1. PERSONAL GOAL-SETTING TABLE				
ROLES	**GOALS**	**ACTION ITEMS**		**STATUS**
		What?	**By When?**	
Active Citizen	Serve on community committee	Identify existing/ existing/proposed committees	7/31/2008	Searching
		Prioritize	8/30/2008	Etc.
		Volunteer	12/31/2008	Etc.
Father	Spend more time with children	read at least one book per week to the children	Now	Starting
Researcher	Have one article published	Submit manuscript to select journals	12/31/2008	Research on-going

- Refer to the lesson for a list of possible entries in the Roles column.

- Just the process of preparing the preceding table can be revealing especially, if at the outset, you have very few rows.

- If you like what you see, such as the possibility of more balance in your life, experiment with the preceding table for at least a month. Update the table weekly and use it to schedule some of your weekly activities. See if your behavior changes and if improved balance is achieved.

Read the following related lessons

- Lesson 3, "Smart Goals"
- Lesson 11, "Afraid of Dying, or Not Having Lived?"
- Lesson 43, "Giving to Our Profession and Our Community"

Study one or more of the following sources cited in this lesson

1. Covey SR. *The 7 Habits of Highly Effective People*. New York: Simon & Schuster; 1990.

2. Brown TL. Time to diversify your life portfolio? *Industry Week*. 1986 (November 10):13.

Refer to one or more of the following supplemental sources

- Rouillard L. Crisp: goals and goal setting. in *Achieving Measured Objectives*. 3rd ed. Menlo Park, CA: Crisp Publications, Inc; 2003. (Provides a step-by-step handbook on how to set goals related to work. Note: You should have your roles identified before using this guide to lay out your goals and measurable outcomes.)

I don't intend to be commonplace.
I intend to make a great person of myself…

great in having fulfilled my possibilities:
great in having seen which of my possibilities are
greatest.

— Arthur Morgan

▫ Lorsch JW, Tierney TJ. Build a life, not a resume. *Consulting to Management.* 2002;(September):44–52. (Offers advice supportive of the roles theme of this lesson. Advocates personal alignment, that is, making decisions that mutually reinforce our "capabilities, goals, needs, and values.")

~~~~~~

All aspects of life are important
And each has its respected legacy.

— James C. McAllister III

Subscribe to one or more of these e-newsletters

▫ "Making a Life, Making a Living" is a monthly e-newsletter produced by Mark S. Albion. Uses questions, humor, quotes and short essays to thoughtfully address a wide variety of personal decision topics. To subscribe, go to http://www.makingalife.com

▫ "The Winner's Circle" is a free e-newsletter provided by the Pacific Institute. Example topics are life strategy, loneliness, goals, coping and parenting. To subscribe, go to http://mailman.wolfe.net/mailman/listinfo/wcn.

~~~~~~

Building an impressive resume
is a lot easier than
building a fulfilling life
because life is a lot more complicated.

— Jay W. Lorsch and Thomas J. Tierney

Lesson 3

Smart Goals

|||||||||||||||||||||||||||||||||||||||||||||||||||||||||||||||||||||||||||||||||||||||

*Those who do not have goals
are doomed to work for those who do.*

— Brian Tracy

The previous lesson titled "Roles, Then Goals" argues that we should decide on our high priority roles (e.g., parent, professional, daughter, friend) before we establish our goals. Why? The danger of establishing goals before defining roles is that we will inadvertently omit or diminish important segments of our being. We risk incurring deep regrets that cannot be remedied. Clear goals, consistent with our selected roles, are crucial to charting and navigating the tumultuous seas of our professional, community and personal life. As stated in the Koran: "If you don't know where you are going, any road will get you there."

As a guide to formulating annual or other goals, consider using the acronym **SMART**.

> *S* means be *S*pecific. A vague goal, such as "become a better member of the pharmacy community" isn't very helpful. Instead try to be more specific such as "become an active member of an ASHP practice section."

M stands for *M*easurable in that, to the extent feasible, each goal should be cast in quantitative terms. An example is "complete 90% of my projects under budget." That which is measurable is more likely to get done.

A refers to *A*chievable. While we should be stretched by goals, we must be able to accomplish each one assuming a sustained, good faith effort. A major goal, such as publishing a journal article, could be broken into ambitious, achievable sub-goals, one of which might be "have an abstract accepted for presentation at a national meeting."

R denotes *R*elevant in that each goal must be relevant to your chosen roles and other constraints. Establishing a goal of starting a service in your hospital that is at odds with the organization's strategy and its business plan fails the relevance test.

T represents *T*ime-framed. Establish a schedule or milestones for achieving a goal or its components.

We are most likely to fulfill our chosen roles if we are guided by well-formulated goals. Are your goals SMART, that is, specific, measurable, achievable, relevant, and time-framed?

Implicit in the preceding advice is that our goals should be written. The suggested SMART technique can only be fully implemented in writing. Conceptualize, refine, and write out monthly, annual and multi-year goals for personal, family, financial, community, and professional areas and affairs.

Having written our goals, we should frequently look at them. Each of us has some control over how we invest some of our time and energy. Important, urgent matters tend to dominate our lives. Working towards goals falls in the important but not urgent category. As such, our goals can wither from lack of attention while we focus our care on urgent demands. We must invest some of our spare moments in reviewing our goals and planning action items to achieve them. The leader in us schedules time to review and refine personal and group goals. Ralph Waldo Emerson, schoolmaster, minister, lecturer and writer said, "Guard your spare moments. They are like uncut diamonds. Discard them and their value will never be known.

Improve them and they will become the brightest gems of a useful life."

A final thought. Selectively share goals with trusted individuals who can help you achieve your objectives. For example, if one of your goals is to work on a particular type of project; discuss the details with your supervisor and others in influential positions. Perhaps you desire to serve on a committee or task force in your department or hospital. Then discuss your interest with appropriate committee chairs, members, or leaders who can help you realize your goal. You are surrounded by people who, if they know you and your goals, will help you achieve them.

*It's never too late to be
what you might have been.*

— George Eliot

Suggestions for Applying Ideas

Write personal SMART goals in each of the following areas for 1 year and 10 years from now

- Annual salary and other compensation.
- Position, such as, project manager, supervisor, coordinator, department manager, or director.
- Functions, such as, recruitment, staff development, inventory control, sales and marketing, compounding, quality improvement initiatives, and general management.
- Other, such as, travel internationally, speak at national meetings, serve in elected office, and publish a paper and/or book.

Identify, for each of the preceding SMART goals, one specific thing you will do this month, for the 1-year goals, and this year, for the 10-year goals

- By setting a goal you are, in effect, "planning a trip." How are you going to get to your destination?
- Do you have the necessary knowledge, skills and attitudes and, if not, a means of obtaining them?

▣ Or are you going to let chance rule perhaps using the rationale that everything will come to you if you "just work hard" and "keep your nose to the grindstone"?

Manage your time wisely, so that you devote sufficient energy to achieving the established SMART goals. Consider these time management ABC's. [1]

▣ Articulate SMART goals—presumably you have already done this.

▣ Plan each day in writing.

▣ Act immediately and constructively. For example, if a communication comes across your desk, immediately act on it, file it or discard it.

~~~~~~~~~~~~~~~~~~~~~~~~~~~~~~~~~~~~

A winner is someone who recognizes his God-given talents,
works his tail off to develop them into skills and
uses these skills to accomplish his goals.

— Larry Bird

▣ Bring at least one potential solution whenever you take a problem to a supervisor, colleague or client. Expect your supervises and others to do the same.

▣ Identify your best time of the day and use it for your most demanding tasks.

▣ Maintain a clean desk and work area to minimize visual distributions.

▣ Create an efficient workspace with frequently used items in easy reach.

▣ Distinguish between efficiency (doings things right) and effectiveness (doing the right things). Both are necessary, but the latter is more important. Goals help us identify the right things.

▣ Create a carefully organized set of hard and/or electronic professional files in which you place potentially useful material for possible future retrieval and use.

- Keep materials for on-going small projects together.
- Meet only when necessary, and, to the extent you have influence, insist that meetings be carefully planned and facilitated.
- Recognize the 20/80 rule of thumb, that is, 20 percent of the input to a process produces 80 percent of the results. Search for and concentrate on input items in the 20 percent.

Devoting a little of yourself to everything
means committing a great deal of yourself to nothing.

— Michael Le Boeuf

- Break large projects into small, manageable—by you or others— parts.
- Use discretionary time wisely, recognizing that time at work may be viewed as falling into one of these three categories: boss-imposed time, system-imposed time, and self-imposed time. Self-imposed time is discretionary time and is most likely to offer opportunities to advance your goals by attending to important but not urgent demands.
- Group similar activities such as returning telephone calls or emails or working on various parts of a report. Grouping tends to be more efficient.
- Avoid "telephone tag" by using techniques such as leaving a specific voice mail message, leaving an intriguing message, suggesting a specific telephone meeting time, and using other forms of communication.
- Delegate appropriate parts of your tasks, along with necessary authority, to other capable individuals.
- Keep "door" closed but access open. You are less likely to be interrupted if your door is closed or the entry to your workspace is

arranged such that potential visitors interrupt only when necessary.

◻ Write it down. Time invested in documentation efforts such as taking notes at a meeting, writing a memorandum to file, or sending an email to meeting participants usually improves understanding of decisions and responsibilities and saves time in the long run.

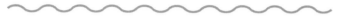

We're lost,
but we're making good time.

— Yogi Berra

◻ Write response on original document. Answer selected hardcopy memoranda and letters by writing a response directly on the document and returning it to the sender, perhaps with copies to others and the file.

◻ Use travel and waiting time productively. Carry small reading or other projects with you along with appropriate tools.

◻ Use word processing, as opposed to writing long hand, but recognize that a handwritten note or card, because of the rarity, can be a very meaningful means of communication.

◻ Meet with yourself, that is, isolate blocks of time during your workday to do tasks requiring higher concentration.

◻ Log your time. Keep a record, at 15- to 30-minute intervals, of how you use your time for several days to a week. Identify and expand productive uses.

◻ Adopt a holistic philosophy by striving for balance among the intellectual, physical, emotional and spiritual dimensions of your life.

◻ Guarantee small successes. Plan each day so it includes one activity that is both enjoyable and likely to be accomplished.

Be prepared to persevere to achieve your more ambitious goals. Consider these examples of perseverance.

◻ Chester Carlson developed the quick electrostatic photography process in the 1940s. This technology was intended to replace the contemporary, cumbersome, copying paradigm which used film, developer, and a darkroom. Incredulously, 43 companies rejected his idea! They passed on the opportunity to develop what is now called xerography and is the basis for the omnipresent copy machines.[2]

- Jeffrey Fudin, a pharmacist employed by the VA, exemplifies the perseverance of a pharmacist to achieve his goal of upholding the Oath of a Pharmacist and to uphold the objectives of the profession of pharmacy in the face of bureaucratic deviance and moral insufficiency when physicians at a VA hospital were accused of performing illegal research on cancer patients.[3]

- Theodor Geisel, more popularly known as Dr. Seuss, is considered a premiere author of children's books. He wrote more than 60 books and, in 1984, won a special Pulitzer Prize. He was a pioneer in linking drawings to text, an approach that appeared in his first book. Within 1 year of writing his first book, it was rejected by 29 publishers before being accepted.[4]

- Joseph B. Strauss, engineer and poet, envisioned a bridge across San Francisco's Golden Gate. In the face of widespread skepticism, including that of his peers, he led the two decade planning, design, and construction of the Golden Gate Bridge. Strauss, who died approximately one year after the May 1937 opening of the bridge, is honored with a statue erected at the south end of the span dedicated to "The Man Who Built the Bridge." The intensity of that effort is suggested by these lines from one of Strauss' poems.[5]

Launched midst a thousand hopes and fears,
dammed by a thousand hostile sneers.
Yet ne'er its course was stayed.
But ask of those who met the foe,
who stood alone when faith was low,
ask them the price they paid.

Unfortunately, Strauss' admirable perseverance was partly offset by his reluctance to acknowledge the contributions of others. For example, Charles A. Ellis, who actually led the design effort, was discharged by an apparently highly egotistical Strauss before construction was completed.[5,6]

~~~~~~~~~~~~~~~~~~~~~~

People are always blaming their circumstances for
what they are.
I don't believe in circumstances.
The people who get on in this world
are the people who get up and look for the circum-
stances they want,
and, if they can't find them, make them.

— George Bernard Shaw

Read the following related lessons

◨ Lesson 2, "Roles, Then Goals"

◨ Lesson 8, "Go Out On a Limb"

◨ Lesson 11, "Afraid of Dying, Or Not Having Lived?"

◨ Lesson 26, "The Power of Our Subconscious"

◨ Lesson 27, "Delegation: Why Put Off Until Tomorrow What Someone Else Can Do Today?"

◨ Lesson 44, "Looking Ahead: Can You Spare a Paradigm?"

Study one or more of the following sources cited in this lesson

1. Walesh SG. "Management of self." In *Engineering Your Future: The Non-Technical Side of Professional Practice In Engineering and Other Technical Fields.* 2nd ed. Reston, VA: ASCE Press; 2000.

2. Barker JA. *Discovering the Future: The Business of Paradigms.* St. Paul, MN: ILI Press; 1989.

3. Fudin J. Blowing the whistle: A pharmacist's vexing experience unraveled. *Am J Health-Syst Pharm.* 2006;63:2262–5.

4. Hurst C. A Collection of Reviews of Children's Books. Available at http://www.carolhurst.com. Accessed July 8, 2007.

5. McGloin JB. Symphonies in steel: Bay Bridge and the Golden Gate. Museum of San Francisco; 2003. Available at http://

www.sfmuseum.org/hist9/mcgloin.html. Accessed July 8, 2007.

6. Fredrich AJ, ed. Strauss gave me some pencils. In *Sons of Martha: Civil Engineering Readings in Modern Literature.* New York: ASCE; 1989.

Refer to one or more of the following supplemental sources

☐ Hensey M. "Setting work, career and personal goals." Chapter 14 in *Personal Success Strategies.* Reston, VA: ASCE Press; 1999.

☐ Hill N. *Think and Grow Rich.* New York: Fawcett Crest; 1960.

☐ Urban H. *Life's Greatest Lesson: 20 Things That Matter.* New York: Simon & Schuster; 2003.

Subscribe to one or more of these e-newsletters

☐ "Personal Achievement Quote of the Day," offered free by the company Top Achievement. Uplifting thoughts from varied accomplished individuals may help you implement your goal-related action plans. To subscribe, go to http://www.topachievement.com/quote.html.

☐ "The Winners Circle Daily Email" is provided free by the Pacific Institute. The Institute and the e-newsletter teach "people how to manage change, set and achieve goals, lead more effectively, and think in ways that create success." To subscribe go to: http://mailman.wolfe.net/mailman/listinfo/wcn.

Visit this website

☐ "Top Achievement" (http://www.topachievement.com/) is the website of the company Top Achievement. Provides many free goal-related articles and access to websites and products.

*You must have long-term goals
to keep you from being frustrated
by short-term failures.*

— Charles Noble

Lesson 4

Experience Excellence

||||||||||||||||||||||||||||||||||||||||||||||||||||||||||||||||||||||||||||||||||||||||||||||||||||||||||

The noblest search is the search for excellence.

— Lyndon B. Johnson

Someone recently told me how competitive they are—with others. This caused me to reflect. I'm competitive, but mostly with myself. I actually believe in the "continuous improvement" mantra of the total quality management movement, but again, focused on me. Incidentally, competition with self is not selfish but rather an attempt to practice good stewardship with one's unique set of gifts.

The most splendid achievement of
all is the constant striving to surpass
yourself and to be worthy of your own approval.

— Dennis Waitley

Reflection immediately after an event or activity, such as leading a webinar, teaching a lecture, holding a staff meeting, completing a project, or solving a problem works for me. Reflection leads to a little improvement here and a little there and, over time, to big improvements. Or, as nicely stated by consultant H. Jackson Brown[1]: "The road to success is not doing one thing 100 percent better, but doing 100 things one percent better."

Another way to compete with—to better—ourselves is to experience excellence exhibited by others. While seeing the superb performance of others may naturally cause some envy, it is much more likely to inspire us; to stimulate us to do whatever we do even better.

Observing how high others have set the bar in their chosen endeavors can cause us to push our bar up another notch. Unfortunately, the opposite is also true. Spending too much time with individuals exhibiting mediocrity and complacency, can tempt us to see our bar as being set high enough or, worse yet, too high and, therefore, convince us to lower it a notch or two.

What is excellence? My dictionary (*Webster's New World*, Third College Edition) defines it as "the fact or condition of excelling; superiority; surpassing goodness." John Gardner, former U.S. Secretary of Health, Education and Welfare, strongly urged us to value excellence in all good things when he said: "The society which scorns excellence in plumbing as a humble activity and tolerates shoddiness in philosophy because it is an exalted activity will have neither good plumbing nor good philosophy: neither its pipes nor its theories will hold water."

To do well in life
we must first think well.

— John C. Maxwell

The following are examples of excellence seen in every day life

- Early in my career, when I was struggling with public speaking, I heard an excellent public speaker. My initial reaction: he was a natural; he was born with that gift. After his presentation he revealed that the opposite was true. His excellent speaking, which appeared so natural, was the result of many years of thoughtful practice. I was inspired to work even harder at my speaking.

▣   My dentist recently performed some restorative work on my teeth. Based on years of experience with him and others, I know that he is expensive, but very good. In this case, I marveled at his skill; how he labored to match color, reproduce pattern, sculpture, shape, and perfect my bite. I was inspired to become even more skillful in what I do.

▣   My wife and I recently attended a play at a small Charleston theater. We were close enough to clearly hear the actors and see their expressions. Although the stage sets were simple, the superb lead performers drew us into the drama repeatedly evoking various emotional responses. The outside world temporarily disappeared. I was inspired to perform even better in my professional endeavor.

▣   And then there was the 2004 Summer Olympics. Setting aside various negative distractions, we experienced excellence many times such as in the swimming of Michael Phelps and the floor exercise of Carly Patterson.

Excellence is doing ordinary things extraordinarily well.

— John W. Gardner

Supplement first hand experiences with people exhibiting excellence by reading or otherwise learning about individuals who have achieved excellence. An excellent way to do this is to skim pharmacy related publications such as *Pharmacy Practice News, Modern Healthcare,* and even the *American Journal of Health-System Pharmacists* on a regular basis looking for articles that describe excellence in practice. A good example of an article you may look for is an article that was recently published in *Pharmacy Practice News*[2] highlighting the efforts of the hospital-wide effort to eradicate ventilator associated pneumonia (VAP). Almost unheard of, the Community Health Network in Indianapolis has had over a 2-year period of VAP free healthcare. This article emphasized that if you reach for excellence and continue to apply efforts towards a goal, you can succeed, and achieve excellence.

Let's proactively expand our activities so that we more frequently experience the excellence scattered all around us. Sometimes it will be costly (e.g., my dentist and the play). Other times we will not have to dig deep; excellence is often nearby and available at little or no cost. Confucius said: "Excellence does not remain alone; it is sure to attract neighbors." Let's seek excellence, including looking for it in our "neighborhood." As a result, someday we will exhibit excellence for others to experience.

Have patience with all things,
but chiefly have patience with yourself.
Do not lose courage in considering your own perfections,
but instantly set about remedying them—
every day begin the task anew.

— St. Francis de Sales

Suggestions for Applying Ideas

Read the following related lessons

- ◻ Lesson 5, "Too Much of a Good Thing"
- ◻ Lesson 8, "Go Out on a Limb"

Study one or more of the following sources cited in this lesson

1. Brown HJ. *A Father's Book of Wisdom.* Nashville, TN: Rutledge Hill Press; 2000.
2. Huff C. Hospitals winning fight vs. ventilator pneumonia. *Pharmacy Practice News.* 2007;34(7):23–5.

Refer to the following supplemental sources

▣ Covey S. *The 7 Habits of Highly Effective People*. New York: Simon and Schuster; 1989.

Stephen Covey describes the 7 habits of personal development which he believes lead to personal growth, realization, and achievement of interdependence. Use these habits to develop an understanding of your self and your goals so that you can achieve them more effectively.

▣ Collins J. *Good to Great*. New York: HarperBusiness; 2001.

Although this book focuses primarily on how to be a competitive and successful leader who is devoted to the success of their organization, applying the hedgehog concept both to self and your organization may be useful.

▣ Levine S. *The Six Fundamentals of Success*. New York: Doubleday; 2004.

This book comprises six fundamentals for organizational success. These fundamentals begin with the individual embrace. Applicable to this lesson is the sixth fundamental "Gain Perspective" which encourages individuals to take time to learn from mistakes and learn how setbacks can make us stronger.

▣ Maxwell JC. *Thinking For a Change: 11 Ways Highly Successful People Approach Life and Work*. New York: Warner Books, Inc; 2003.

Focuses on 11 different thinking skills to channel and harness your motivation to succeed and achieve excellence. It shows you how to think in different ways to challenge yourself to go the places and achieve the goals you've always wanted to complete.

The foundation of lasting self-confidence
and self esteem is excellence, mastery of your work.

— Brian Tracey

Visit the following website

- "Personal Development.com" (http://www.personal-development.com) provides self-improvement articles, resources and a free newsletter that assist individuals achieve excellence.

Too Much of a Good Thing

|||||||||||||||||||||||||||||||||||||||||||||||||||||||||||||||||||||||||||||||||||||||||||

The trouble with experience is that by the time you have it you are too old to take advantage of it.

— Jimmy Connors

A downturn in the stock market as indicated, for example, by a sharp drop in the Dow Jones Industrial Average, is disconcerting for many of us. Suddenly retirement accounts, mutual funds, and other investments plummet in value. Our net worth drops sharply. There is the gnawing fear of the negative long-term effect on the material well being of our spouse and dependents. We vow to be even more watchful of our investments. After all, prudence requires careful management of personal financial assets.

What about the status of and attention to personal professional assets? Although the value of our professional assets defies quantification, it is nevertheless very real. The quality of our experience is a major part of those assets. Experience gives us the ability and confidence to take on new challenges, including more managing and leading. Thoughtfully applied, experience also helps us learn from and not repeat mistakes. Nevertheless, someone has pessimistically said "experience is wonderful, it helps us recognize a mistake the second time we make it" and, somewhat more positively, consider this definition: experience is what we get when we don't get what we wanted.

While experience is valuable, too much of one kind of experience can hamper individual growth. Accordingly, each of us should appraise his or her professional assets at least once a year, in part to assess the quality of and freshness of our experience. Ask yourself "What specific actions did you have for your own professional growth?"

Many people end up in the wrong place
only because they stayed in the right place too long

— John C. Maxwell

This evaluation of professional assets might be in the form of a resume update exercise. What new areas of technology have been mastered? What new management and leadership techniques were used? What new concepts, ideas, or principles were studied? How has our attitude improved? What new skills were acquired? What new challenges and responsibilities were accepted? What new opportunities were seized and new risks were taken? What knowledge was shared with co-workers and others? What new contributions were made? In what ways have we been "good and faithful servants" with our talents?

As we review several annual accountings of our professional experience, will we find several years each filled with new experiences? Or will we find 1 year of experience repeated several times? If the latter is true, we may be in the midst of a devastating professional assets "stock market crash."

The value of professional assets, if approximated by the present worth of one's future income, will greatly exceed the value of a younger person's net worth, except for those fortunate few who are independently wealthy. Like personal financial assets, personal professional assets can appreciate, plateau, or decline.

We should resist the temptation to settle into the comfort of routine, rationalizing it in the name of gaining more experience. Author and lecturer, Og Mandino, in his book *The Greatest Salesman in the World*, offers this warning about excessive experience[1] :

> I will commence my journey unencumbered with either the weight of unnecessary knowledge or the handicap of meaningless experience. In truth, experience teaches thoroughly yet her course of instruction devours men's years so the value of her lessons diminishes with the time necessary to acquire her special wisdom.

The "I need more experience before ..." position often reflects a sincere desire to be properly prepared before taking on a new task, function or other challenge. In some cases, the claim that more experience is needed reflects deep-seated fear of advancement; it becomes a rationalization for staying put. Clearly, as suggested by Mandino's advice, we need to strike a balance between too little and too much experience. Using a sailing metaphor, author Richard Bode gives this advice for achieving balance[2]:

> The frantic individual tacks too soon, jumping from job to job. The obtuse individual remains on the same tack too long, investing too much time, talent, and energy in a course that takes him far from his avowed objectives. But the seasoned sailor stays on the same tack as long as it appears advantageous, and then deftly changes directions. The confirmed sailor goes on tacking forever.

Each of us has opportunities to deftly change direction so that we gain new and valuable professional experience. Examples of ways to acquire asset-building management and leadership experience include asking for new job assignments, requesting a transfer to another part of our organization, seeking a new employer, returning to school, establishing our own business, and becoming active in a professional or business organization. In the final analysis, each of us has his or her hand on the tiller.

The ultimate determinant of our progress is the strength and persistence of will of each individual practitioner

— Paul G. Pierpaoli

Suggestions for Applying Ideas

Apply the Shewart Cycle[3] as a means of maximizing what you learn from experiences

- The Shewart Cycle is the plan-do-study-act process of continuous improvement:
  - Plan a step or steps toward a goal,
  - Do as per the plan,
  - Study the results, and
  - Act to improve the step or steps and repeat the cycle.

- The value of applying the Shewart Cycle to experience is that it emphasizes the need to examine our experiences. Experience per se is of no value. We must examine our experiences to avoid missing opportunities to learn. Rather than repeatedly having the same experience, or kind of experience, the Shewart Cycle helps us benefit from our experience and, therefore move on to different and higher level experiences.

- Consider a professional experience you are about to have. Examples might be leading a project, training a new employee, interviewing for a new position, giving a talk, and attending a meeting. Consciously apply the Shewart Cycle as follows:
  - Plan the experience, at least the aspects you control or influence,
  - Do, that is, carry out the plan,
  - Study, and learn from, the results, and
  - Act, that is decide what you would do the same and differently the next time, and then do it that way when the opportunity arises.

Prove to your own satisfaction,

that every adversity, failure, defeat, sorrow

and unpleasant circumstance,

whether of your own making or otherwise,

carries with it the seed of an equivalent benefit

which may be transmitted into a

blessing of great proportions.

— Napoleon Hill

Look to your immediate surroundings for new profession-related experience opportunities

Someone in a professional rut may prematurely decide that new experiences require a new employer. While the grass may be greener on the other side of the fence, green patches may already lie on your side. Consider these possibilities within your current employment situation:

- ☒ Share some or all of your goals with a supervisor and ask for a challenging assignment consistent with one or more of your goals.

- ☒ Request a transfer to or apply for a position in another department, office, or other organizational unit. Or, even another position within your department of pharmacy may better meet your needs. Even if financial compensation remains the same, the range and variety of experiences is likely to grow and eventually lead to more opportunities and increased compensation.

- ☒ Offer to accompany others who are attending meetings, participating in projects, and carrying out other functions. Vicariously experience their decision-making, presentations, discussions, and other actions.

In the business world,
everyone is paid in two coins:
cash and experience.
Take the experience first;
the cash will come later.

— Harold Geneen

Consider the similarity between learning from experience and digesting food[4]

- Our bodies extract nourishment from food, even when we don't eat well, and eliminate what is not needed.

- Similarly, we can learn to extract knowledge from our positive and negative experiences and let go of the residue, that is, whatever does not serve us.

Where we go from here will depend largely on our
ability to continue to learn…and to change.

— Grover C. Bowles

Read the following related lessons

- Lesson 9, "Keeping Our Personal Financial Score"
- Lesson 13, "So What Do You Know About Macaws?"

Study one or more of the following sources cited in this lesson

1. Mandino O. *The Greatest Salesman in The World.* New York: Bantam Books; 1968.

2. Bode R. *First You Have to Row a Little Boat.* New York: Warren Books; 1993.

3. Hensey M. Learning how to learn. Chapter 6 in *Personal Success Strategies.* Reston, VA: ASCE Press; 1999.

4. Chopra D, Simon D. *Grow Younger, Live Longer: 10 Steps to Reverse Aging.* New York: Three Rivers Press; 2002.

Refer to the following supplemental source

◘ Hill N. *Think and Grow Rich.* New York, NY: Fawcett Crest; 1960. (Reports on a 25-year study of the experiences of highly accomplished individuals. Concludes that the common element is the power of visualization—looking way beyond one's current situation—linked with the subconscious mind.)

~~~~~~~~~~~~~~~~~~~~~~

From time to time,
everyone benefits from being "re-potted,"
from applying their talents to new challenges.
Re-potting and self-renewal go hand in hand,
whether the pot is a new position, a new firm,
or an entirely new career.

— Jay W. Lorsch and Thomas J. Tierney

Lesson 6

DWYSYWD

||||||||||||||||||||||||||||||||||||||||||||||||||||||||||||||||||||||||||||||||||||||

It is better that you should not vow than that you should vow and not pay.

— Ecclesiastes 5:5, Bible, Revised Standard Version

Promises punctuate our professional and private lives. They are mostly small, with big ones intermingled, but nevertheless all are promises— or at least seem to be. We could easily hear a dozen or more promises on any given day. However, informed by experience, we gradually learn that there are "promises" and there are promises. The former are just words and the latter are commitments to action; are as good as done.

One way we risk engendering mistrust, tarnishing our reputations, and frustrating our aspirations, is by failing to keep small promises. For example, you meet someone at a local meeting of a professional society. You exchange business cards and promise to send them a copy of a collaborative practice agreement to help them build their practice. But you forget. Or you run into an acquaintance that you have not seen for some time, talk briefly, and agree you and he should get together for lunch. You offer to make arrangements. But you forget. Other examples of promises, often not kept:

◘ *I'll send* you a copy of the material.

◘ Send me the draft report; *I'll give* you my comments.

◘ *I'll draft* the minutes; you will have them within three days.

◘ Don't worry about correcting this order, *I'll do* it.

◘ *I'll contact* the Department of Pharmacy regarding this matter and get back to you.

Breaking promises like those cited here might be considered insignificant oversights. But are they harmless, especially if part of a pattern?

We might argue that breaking small promises is not a significant issue. Small promises are in the gray area, you say. Perhaps. After all, there are no explicit "small promises" canons, rules, principles, or tenets in the various ethics codes governing professional practice of pharmacy. The immediate consequence of any unfilled small promise, such as not attending a meeting, forgetting to send an e-mail, or missing lunch, is usually small. Furthermore, pharmacy is built on a foundation of medicine, patient care and more recently technology. Small, interpersonal failings would pale in importance to such matters as medicine based patient care or technology implementation.

However, having opportunities to effectively perform our duties as pharmacists and pharmacy leaders requires developing a web of mutually trustful relationships with co-workers, physicians, nurses, administrators, regulators, and others. Clearly, major transgressions are likely to permanently shatter trust or prevent it from occurring. However, and this is the point of this lesson, cumulative small lapses can have the same effect. They gradually exclude us from the web of those who have faith and confidence in each other and we miss managing and leading opportunities.

Those who routinely don't do what they say they will do are sometimes creative and well-intentioned. However, these positive qualities do not lead, as they could, to positive outcomes because the creative, well-intentioned individuals are poor managers of their personal time and affairs. They lack the discipline to write down, in hard copy or electronically, their promises and periodically review and act on their "to do" list. As a result those they interact with miss out on the fruits of creative thoughts.

Others who don't do what they said they would do make promises because they become entrapped, in knee jerk fashion, by a desire to please. They promise because it seems to be the thing to do. They haven't learned how to say no or to say nothing. Their promises are shallow and lack conviction.

If someone throws you a ball,
you don't have to catch it.

— Richard Carlson

Regardless of the reasons for frequently not following through on promises, which can be many and varied, the fate of those who don't is common: loss of credibility. Family, friends, colleagues, clients, potential clients and others gradually recognize the wide gulf between what the person "promises" and what he or she delivers. We are increasingly reluctant to rely on certain individuals and may "write off" others after concluding that their promises, regardless of motivation, are just vibrations in the air. To the extent feasible, we avoid entanglements in their webs.

Talk is cheap to some of the people we encounter as evidenced by the lavish way they dispense words. Enthusiasm abounds, ideas flow, proposals are presented and promises are made. However, experience with these individuals gradually reveals that promises, big and small, are not kept. While we may continue contact with the "talkers," they are not likely to be part of our trusted circle of colleagues. We begin to question their management competency and leadership potential.

Successful implementation of a project or roll-out of a new hospital-wide practice requires careful planning, designing, and strategic implementation. The amount of time one task takes or the amount of debate about a specific detail doesn't necessarily determine its importance. Even the smallest aspect or piece of a project can have a large impact on the outcome. Recall the innocuous O-rings that precipitated the Challenger disaster or from a pharmacy perspective, failure of intravenous infusion devices due to battery failures. Similarly, successful development of mutually trustful relationships demands attention to both the big picture and the little details. Trust is built piece-by-piece; some pieces are large but many are small. By keeping small promises, we build big relationships.

We pharmacists should do whatever is necessary to earn and retain patient, customer, citizen, and other stakeholder trust. Keeping promises, including little ones, is essential to trustful relationships. My advice: DWYSYWD, that is, do what you said you would do.

No virtue is more universally accepted
as a test of good character
than trustworthiness.

— Harry Emerson Fosdick

Suggestions for Applying Ideas

Follow up immediately and, if possible, in writing, on each promise

- If you met with someone and promised to send them a document, draft a memorandum or email and/or obtain the documents as soon as you get back to your office. The point: do something to start the process of following through on your promise.

- If you promised to arrange a meeting with someone, place a reminder in your time management system to contact that person. Make the entry in that person's presence; it suggests your commitment.

Do what you said you were going to do,
when you said you were going to do it,
and how you said you were going to do it.

— Byrd Baggett

Consider this advice on promise making from Robert Townsend,[1] the blunt speaking former CEO of the Avis car rental company

- If asked when you can deliver something, ask for time to think.
- Build in a margin of safety.
- Name a date.
- Then deliver it earlier than you promised.
- He concludes his advice by saying "The world is divided into two classes of people: the few who make good on their promises (even if they don't promise as much), and the many who don't."

Read the following related lesson

Lesson 3, "Smart Goals" (the time management portion)

Study the following source cited in this lesson

1. Townsend R. *Up the Organization: How to Stop the Corporation from Stifling People and Strangling Profits.* New York: Alfred A. Knopf; 1970.

You cannot live on other people's promises,
but if you promise others enough,
you can live on your own.

— Mark Caine

Courage: Real and Counterfeit

||||||||||||||||||||||||||||||||||||||||||||||||||||||||||||||||||||||||||||||||||||||||

*It is curious that physical courage
should be so common in the world
and moral courage so rare.*

— Mark Twain

Leadership and significant achievement require courage—courage to set high personal and group goals, to keep the faith in the face of major set-backs, to hold people accountable for carrying out their responsibilities and keeping their promises, to confront individuals exhibiting unacceptable behavior, to walk away from a project on ethical grounds, to aim high and risk apparent great failure, to apologize and ask for a second chance, and to persist when all others have given up. But, what constitutes courage and courageous people? The aspiring leader that lies within many of us would like to know.

The Greek philosopher Aristotle[1] offers a thoughtful and demanding perspective on courage. He defines courage as a precarious, difficult-to-prescribe balance between causes, motives, means, timing, and confidence. Aristotle says:

The man, then, who faces and who fears the right things and from the right motive, in the right way and at the right time, and who feels confidence under the corresponding conditions, is brave; for the brave man feels and acts according to the merits of the case and in whatever way the rule directs.

Aristotle goes on to say that courage is a mean between cowardice and rashness, confidence and fear. In summary, he defines courage as a fully informed, carefully considered willingness to die for a noble cause. Aristotle refutes the notion that courage is reactive or instinctive. We might be tempted to say that Aristotle was not totally serious about his definitions of courage and courageous people—at least with respect to the "willingness to die" aspect. After all, he must have intended death as a metaphor for a willingness to incur great loss. This interpretation is probably acceptable.

Aristotle outlines in systematic and exhaustive fashion five kinds of false courage. These might be referred to as lesser degrees of courage. They encompass much of what passes for courage in our society and help, by elimination, to define bona fide courage.

- The first type of courage is *coercion courage* or what Aristotle refers to as "the courage of the citizen-soldier." The possessor faces significant risks, but he or she has no choice. Leaders simply have to do many things—some of which are quite unpleasant and risky. Aristotle's coercion courage concept cautions the leader in us to maintain perspective and not to view these as courageous acts worthy of praise. These acts are part of the job; they come with the territory.

- What might be called high information or *calculated courage* is the second type. Aristotle uses the example of the professional soldier who seems brave in battle, but in fact entered the fray with far superior information and other resources that virtually guaranteed victory. According to World War II air ace Eddie Rickenbacker, "courage is doing what you're afraid to do. There can be no courage unless you're scared." The leader in us may be tempted to feign courage because we have exclusive access to vital information.

~~~~~~

It is easy to be brave from a safe distance

— Aesop

▢ The third type of courage is ***passion courage***. These reactionary acts conflict with the choice and motive elements clearly evident in Aristotle's model of courage. While the emotional outburst or sharp retort is often viewed as courage—as in "you sure told him/her"—these acts are often done without thought. Although passionate reactions seem to immediately please some onlookers, calm and reason in difficult circumstances may require more courage and lead to greater long-term benefits for all antagonists.

▢ Sanguine, to use Aristotle's word, or what might be called ***overly optimistic courage***, is the fourth type of counterfeit courage. A string of business or other successes can lead to unrealistic optimism or even complacency, which may be viewed as courage. The U.S. global dominance in economic and military affairs during the four-decade post-World War II period is an illustration of Aristotle's sanguine courage. The modern leader must be alert and view expectations of continued success with suspicion. An earlier atmosphere of courage that enables an organization to achieve high levels of performance may gradually and unnoticeably give way to complacency.

~~~~~~

Pharmacists must have character and courage,
more essential than ever because the corporate stakes
and corporate influences in pharmacy have escalated,
and require unquestionable moral compass.

— Billy W. Woodward

▢ Aristotle's fifth type of false courage is the ***ignorance variety***. As he bluntly says, "people who are ignorant of the danger also appear brave." As we become an increasingly information-rich world, the leader in us must devote appropriate resources to continuously sifting through new knowledge to identify and assess opportunities and threats. At any given time, our courage may, in fact, be based on a lack of data and information describing the dire circumstances we are facing.

Informed by Aristotle's ideas, the aspiring leader in each of us is more likely to recognize our and others' bravado. There will always be some pretense of bravery—particularly by people in high and prestigious positions. Recognizing this, the leader should place a premium on his or her acts and the acts of others that, in the face of risk and calamity, are carefully considered and indicate a willingness to sacrifice for the corporate or community cause. Courageous acts don't have to be extreme acts. When leaders take extreme positions, they may be less successful in defending a principle, advancing a cause, or achieving a worthy goal than when they assume courageous, but somewhat more moderate postures. The leader in each of us recognizes various types of false courage and seeks instead a courage that balances causes, motives, means, timing, and confidence.

Far better it is to dare mighty things,
to win glorious triumphs,
even though checkered by failure,
than to take rank with those poor spirits
who neither enjoy much nor suffer much,
because they live in the gray twilight
that knows not victory nor defeat.

— Theodore Roosevelt

Suggestions for Applying Ideas

Try something very new in your professional or personal life

☐ Think of one or more potentially valuable tasks or actions that you have long wanted to take on or do but, frankly, did not act on because of fear. Possible examples drawn from professional work environment are mentoring a pharmacy student or resident, speaking at a major conference, managing a large project, and leading a department.

☐ Informed by Aristotle's balanced definition of courage and his call for commitment, develop an action plan to do that which you have, until now, feared to do.

☐ Implement your plan in a step-by-step manner.

Do not follow where the path may lead.
Go instead where there is no path
and leave a trail.

— Anonymous

Read the following related lessons

☐ Lesson 8, "Go Out on a Limb"

☐ Lesson 11, "Afraid of Dying, or Not Having Lived?"

☐ Lesson 44, "Looking Ahead: Can You Spare a Paradigm?

Study the following source cited in this lesson

1. Aristotle. *The Nicomachean Ethics*. Translated by D. Ross and revised by J.L. Ackrill and J.O. Urmson. Oxford: Oxford University Press; 1987.

To sin by silence,
when they should protest
makes cowards of men.

— Abraham Lincoln

Lesson 8

Go Out on a Limb

|||||||||||||||||||||||||||||||||||||||||||||||||||||||||||||||||||||||||||||||||||||

Don't be afraid to go out on a limb.
That's where the fruit is.

— Anonymous

In our professional lives, we pharmacists and other clinical professionals tend to be prudent, systematic, and risk averse. Given the great impact of much of our work on patient safety, health, and welfare our overriding caution is warranted. However, we should occasionally do something impulsive, unplanned, and risky. Look over the top of our silo. Leap before we look. Take a shot in the dark. Think outside of the box.

What specific actions do you have
for your own personal growth?

— John W. Webb

Why? Because by doing so we are likely to discover something new and valuable about ourselves while opening doors of opportunity for ourselves, others and our organizations. Frances Bacon, the English philosopher and statesman, put it this way: "A wise man will make more opportunities then he finds." Going out on a limb is a powerful means of encountering opportunities. Even if we do not find an opportunity, we will find out more about ourselves.

If you are introverted and shy, remember that many professional actors share this trait. However, they have learned an important principle: "just say the lines." You can apply this advice.

Our life is in play, the clock is running. There are no time outs, although there may be a two-minute warning. If life is becoming humdrum and work is getting boring, maybe we need to try a completely different ploy, a risky plan—perhaps a "Hail Mary." The status quo, or minor variations on it, won't do. As someone wisely, but anonymously said, "If you do what you always did, you'll get what you always got."

Let's be our sane and safe selves most of the time. But, every now and then, go out on a limb; that's where the best fruit may be.

Security is a false god;
begin making sacrifices to it and you are lost.

— Paul Bowles

Suggestions for Applying Ideas

"Go out on a limb" in your professional, community or personal life

Because going out on a limb is so individual and circumstance specific, meaningful examples are difficult to present. However, for illustration purposes, consider the following, all of which are based on actual situations:

- Contact your local or regional newspaper, television or radio station. Explain that you are an expert in XYZ (e.g., medication safety) and are available to be of assistance to reporters. Nothing may come of your offer, but, on the other hand, you may become the regional XYZ expert!

▣ Think of a prestigious or otherwise desirable organization that you would like to serve as a consultant or an employee. Call a decision-maker at that organization, tell them of your desire to serve or be employed and why. Nothing may happen, but, on the other hand, you may become engaged with the organization or new employer.

▣ Identify a controversial issue in your area of specialty about which you have a strong, informed opinion. Submit a thought-provoking letter to the editor of a widely read journal, magazine or newspaper. Nothing may happen, but, on the other hand, a series of enlightening follow-up letters may appear and you may meet some interesting and powerful people. You may be surprised with the number and variety of people who "come out of the woodwork" as a result of publication of your views.

Things may come to those who wait,
but only the things left by those who hustle.

— Abraham Lincoln

▣ Pick up a newsletter or journal completely outside of pharmacy. As you read it, look for articles or news items having apparent connections or overlaps to what you do or know a lot about. Contact the authors/editors and note the similarities between their work and yours. Nothing may come of it but, on the other hand, you may gain new insight and expand your network.

▣ Approach a person in your field whom you sincerely believe is highly regarded and is powerful. Explain that you are starting out or are striving to advance and would value their advice. Depending on the physical and other circumstances, offer to "buy lunch," telephone them at their convenience, or communicate by email. Be prepared with a list of five to ten concerns you have or questions you'd like to ask. Nothing may happen but, on the other hand, you may acquire a valuable coach or even mentor.

■ If you have basic teaching ability and desire, and possess a body of knowledge and experience to share, contact the continuing education/training chapter of an appropriate professional/business/education organization and offer your services (gratis or for a fee plus expenses). Taking this one step further, or going farther out on a limb, plan, advertise, conduct and follow up on your own seminar/workshop at a hotel/conference center. Nothing may happen but, on the other hand, you may have successful seminars and make many valuable contacts. The "worst" outcome is that you and possibly others incur expenses and the event is cancelled for lack of registrants, but even then your name and services have been exposed to hundreds or thousands of people whom you may work with in the future.

Those who take bold chances
don't think failure is the opposite of success.
They believe that complacency is.

— Richard Farson

■ Call a political or other leader in your community or state. Offer your expertise for service on a committee or board. Nothing may happen, but, on the other hand, you may be asked to participate in or lead an exciting new venture.

Read the following related lessons

■ Lesson 7, "Courage: Real and Counterfeit"
■ Lesson 11, "Afraid of Dying, or Not Having Lived?"

There is a tide in the affairs of men,
which, taken at the flood, leads onto fortune;
omitted, all the voyage of their life is bound in the
shallows and miseries.
On such a full sea are we now afloat;
and we must take the current when it serves or lose
our ventures.

— Shakespeare

Lesson 9

Keeping Our Personal Financial Score

|||||||||||||||||||||||||||||||||||||||||||||||||||||||||||||||||||||||||||||||||||||||

Plan ahead:
It wasn't raining
when Noah built the ark.

— Richard Cushing

Most of us who participate in sports like running, tennis, and golf keep score. We do this partly to determine who won the particular race, match, or round. From a broader perspective, especially if we participate in the sport over a period of years, we keep score to determine our progress. That is, are we improving, have we plateaued, or are we sliding backward?

In a similar fashion, keeping score applies to our personal (or family) financial "game." That is, how have we performed financially and what does past performance predict about our future performance?

We may be tempted to use annual earnings as a surrogate measure of our personal financial score. For example, you note that your annual income this year is 5% more than last year and conclude that you are doing just fine. I am reminded of an acquaintance who said, "Expenses rise to meet anticipated income." Given that most of us have the ability to spend in an almost unlimited fashion, using annual income as a gauge of personal financial success leaves a lot to be desired.

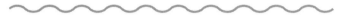

Your income does not determine your outcome.

— Charles J. Givens

A much better measure is net worth which is defined as assets minus liabilities. The tool for determining our net worth is the balance sheet. If we own or owe anything, we have the basis for constructing a balance sheet.

Consider using spreadsheet software for creating your balance sheet. List, in rows, all of your assets (e.g., value of residence, mutual funds, and retirement accounts) and all your liabilities (e.g., balance due on residence, credit cards, and college loans). Use columns to represent the end of each year. Calculate total assets, total liabilities and net worth by year. Update the balance sheet at least annually and save the data from previous years so that you build a personal financial history.

We will derive at least two benefits from maintaining a personal balance sheet. First, it provides ready access to the asset and liability data required by banks and other lending institutions in support of applications for home mortgages, automobile loans, and other common financial transactions. Second, and this is the principal point of this lesson, we can track the "score" of our personal financial "game." Are we building net worth, plateauing, or sliding backwards?

Even if we are building net worth, are we doing it fast enough to meet the financial needs consistent with our retirement and other goals? For example, assume you and your partner are each 30 years old and have a total annual after tax income of $90,000. You want to retire completely at age 62 and, at that time, have an annual income equal to one and one half times the buying power of today's income. Further assume that inflation will average three percent between now and then and you plan to live off of your net worth at age 62 by means of it yielding and growing at a rate of seven percent per year. That is, you want your net worth to remain constant after age 62. Given the preceding assumptions, you will need to accumulate, by age 62, a net worth of $4.9 million.

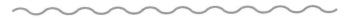

He who will not economize
will have to agonize.

— Confucius

Is your net worth increasing? Is the rate sufficient to provide the financial resources to support your retirement and other goals? Keeping your personal financial "score" will help you answer these questions and, more importantly, take necessary corrective actions. Keeping our financial score puts us in the driver's seat. As succinctly stated by investment banker Roger W. Babson, "Most people should learn to tell their dollars where to go instead of asking them where they went." We must steer our dollars rather than allowing them to steer us.

Suggestions for Applying Ideas

Create a personal balance sheet

■ Possibly using the format in Table 9–1.[1]

Forecast the net worth you will need at retirement

■ Possibly using the procedure in Table 9–2.

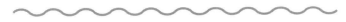

You can create far more wealth
by how you use the money you already earn
than you can from earning more.

— Charles J. Givens

TABLE 9-1. SAMPLE PERSONAL BALANCE SHEET			
	VALUE ($)		
ASSETS	**This Year**	**Last Year**	**Etc.**
House/condominium			
Vehicle(s)			
Stocks/bonds			
Retirement accounts (e.g., IRAs)			
Money market			
Checking account			
Insurance cash value			
Other			
Total:			
LIABILITIES			
Mortgages			
Other loans			
Credit cards			
Other			
Total:			
NET WORTH			
INCREASE IN NET WORTH (%)			

TABLE 9-2. SAMPLE PERSONAL NET WORTH STATEMENT		
FACTOR	**EXAMPLE**	**YOU**
Current age	30	
Current income ($)	90,000	
Desired retirement age	62	
Years until retirement	32	
Expected annual inflation (%)	3	
Current income adjusted for inflation at retirement ($)	$(90,000)(1.03)^{32} =$ 231,750	
Desired ratio of buying power at retirement to buying power now	1.5	
Income required at retirement ($)	$(231,750)(1.5) =$ 347,625	
Annual yield of net worth at retirement (%)	7	
NET WORTH REQUIRED AT RETIREMENT ($)	$(347,625)/(0.07) =$ $4,966,071	

Compare your financial related characteristics to the following "seven common denominators among those who successfully build wealth"

This list is based on a study of American millionaires by author, lecturer and researcher Thomas J. Stanley and marketing professor William D. Danko:[1]

- ◘ They live well below their means.
- ◘ They allocate their time, energy and money efficiently, in ways conducive to building wealth.
- ◘ They believe financial independence is more important than displaying high social status.
- ◘ Their parents did not provide economic outpatient care.
- ◘ Their adult children are economically self-sufficient.
- ◘ They are proficient in targeting market opportunities.
- ◘ They chose the right occupation.

Consistent with this lesson, the authors of the cited study, precisely define wealth. Wealth is not the same as income. If you make a good income each year and spend it all, you are not getting wealthier. You are just living high. Wealth is what you accumulate, not what you spend.

Read the following related lessons

- ◘ Lesson 2, "Roles, Then Goals"
- ◘ Lesson 3, "Smart Goals"
- ◘ Lesson 11, "Afraid of Dying, or Not Having Lived?"
- ◘ Lesson 44, "Looking Ahead: Can You Spare a Paradigm?"

Study one or more of the following sources cited in this lesson

1. Stanley TJ, Danko WD. *The Millionaire Next Door.* New York: Pocket Books; 1996.

Refer to one or more of the following supplemental sources

◻ Belsky G, Gilovich T. *Why Smart People Make Big Money Mistakes – And How to Correct Them.* New York: Simon & Schuster; 1999.

Motivates us to think about behavioral economics which explains why we sometimes make illogical decisions that adversely affect our financial well being. For example, is one of the following two decisions more prudent and, if so, which one: saving $25 on a $200 purchase or saving $25 on a $2000 purchase? Really? Read this book to learn the answer and to learn more about useful topics including the power of compounding, accounting for inflation, the sunk cost fallacy and mental accounting.

◻ Handy, C. *The Hungry Spirit: Beyond Capitalism: A Quest for Purpose in the Modern World.* New York: Broadway Books. 1998.

Recognizes the importance of financial well-being but notes that "money is the means of life and not the point of it." Advocates "proper selfishness" which is defined as accepting "responsibility for making the most of oneself by, ultimately, finding a purpose beyond and bigger than oneself."

◻ Kiyosaki RT, Lechter SL. *Rich Dad, Poor Dad: What the Rich Teach Their Kids About Money—That the Poor and Middle Class Do Not!* New York: Warner Books; 1998.

Stresses the importance of financial literacy, notes that it is not taught in school, and stresses the need to teach and learn financial literacy at home and/or on our own. Numerous asset building ideas and tips are offered.

Almost any man knows how to earn money,
but not one in a million knows how to spend it.

— Henry David Thoreau

Visit one or more of these websites

◻ "Kiplinger.com" (http://www.kiplinger.com) is the website of The Kiplinger Washington Editors, Inc. Included are calculators to assist with financial planning and decisions such as determining net worth, estimating the cost of raising a child and saving for college.

◻ "MSN Money" (http://moneycentral.msn.com/home.asp) includes practical advice on the elements of financial planning such as retirement needs, debt management, and insurance.

◻ "Smartmoney" (http://www.smartmoney.com/pf/) is the website of *Smart Money* magazine. Includes financial planning worksheets and calculators.

Some know the price of everything
and the value of nothing.

— Anonymous

Job Security is an Oxymoron;
Career Security Doesn't Have to Be

||||||||||||||||||||||||||||||||||||||||||||||||||||||||||||||||||||||||||||||||||||||

I must create a system
or be enslaved by another man's.

— William Blake

Throughout the hard times of the Great Depression if you were lucky enough to have a job, you did everything you could to keep it. People understood the importance of job security. A decade after the Depression, the U.S. was in World War II, and a decade later our country was a global economic leader.[1] The secure jobs that were so highly valued during the Great Depression had become commonplace. Workers and employers entered into informal agreements whereby workers gave a day's work for a day's pay and the employer provided a secure job. To show employer appreciation for their loyalty and confirm the job security which was intrinsic in their jobs, workers often received gold watches after 25 years of service.

Today gold watches, and the job security they represented, are rare. Job security, which may be defined as knowing you will be allowed to do the same thing at the same place for a long time, is an oxymoron. Job security passed away because of increased personal productivity, global competition, outsourcing, privatization, reengineering, and consolidation of organizations.

~~~~~~

Job security is gone.
The driving force of a career
must come from the individual.

— Homa Bahrami

However, there is good news! Enlightened clinical professionals who carefully manage their careers can thrive in the new world of work. They can enjoy career security, that is, knowing they will always be employable somewhere and having fun, success, and satisfaction in the process. Guaranteed employment with one organization is out; guaranteed employability is a viable replacement.[2]

~~~~~~

If money is your hope for independence
you will never have it.
The only real security
that a man can have in this world
is a reserve of knowledge, experience, and ability.

— Henry Ford

Thriving in today's economy requires each of us, as an employee, to think, plan, and perform as though we were on our own, or an independent economic unit. Offered here are six suggestions for earning career security as a pharmacist in the modern work world. Each career security suggestion is developed further in the applications portion of this lesson.

   ◻ ***Protect your reputation.*** A pharmacist usually provides clinical
      services in the form of a patient-related outcome, not a material

product. The credibility imparted to those clinical services is closely tied to the professional's reputation. Patients may not able to accurately judge the quality of the information provided to them, or the healthcare they receive. However, the client is quite capable of judging the quality of the professional based on facts or perceptions.

▣ ***Attend to personal and professional development.*** Another aspect of thriving in today's professional market is creating and implementing an ambitious personal and professional development plan. Some employers expect us to plan our personal and professional development and help us with it; however, such employers are rare. Clearly, in the face of such organizational indifference, you must take the lead. Don't expect your employer to "take care of" your development.

▣ ***Invest a dime of every dollar.*** Invest at least ten percent of your earnings beginning with the first dollar on your first job and extending throughout your career. Leverage your investments by taking full advantage of employer and government sponsored programs that match your investments and shield your investments, and the earnings on them, from income taxes.

Security isn't securities.
It's knowing that someone cares
whether you are or cease to be.

— Malcolm Forbes

▣ ***Enhance communication competence.*** Effective communication is necessary, although not sufficient, to realizing your potential. Unless you are a genius, are inextricably linked to business ownership, or enjoy some other rare privilege, you will need effective communication skills to earn career security. Listening, speaking, writing, use of visuals and application of clinical, business and pharmaceutical knowledge are the five pivotal communication skills needed by the professional pharmacist.

■ *Cultivate contacts.* The current term for cultivating contacts is networking. Although it is well known that there is a "shortage" of pharmacists, staying connected to the pharmacist network, and making connections with fellow colleagues is imperative to staying up to date on career and collaboration opportunities. Many job positions are posted in pharmacy journals, and on organization websites (such as ASHP, ACCP, and APhA) but having a personal connection with an employer may enhance the relationship and potential employment eligibility with that employer. Frequently, even with the pharmacist "shortage," job positions may be posted to the public, but will be offered to either internal candidates or candidates with which there is an already established relationship, making the application process very competitive for external candidates who have not stayed in the network of pharmacists.

The demise of job security is a positive development for the profession of pharmacy. It is stimulating growth of a subgroup of independent, entrepreneurial, "on top" rather than "on tap" pharmacists and other clinical professionals who have earned career security. We can join that group by practicing an enlightened selfishness intended to optimize our potential to be faithful stewards of the gifts we've been given. There are only two futures for any of us; the one we create for ourselves or the one others create for us.

Suggestions for Applying Ideas

Consider these thoughts on protecting our reputations

■ Our reputation is what colleagues, clients, and others really "hear" and "see" when we speak, write, or otherwise interact with them. Guard that reputation as though it were your most valued asset; it probably is.

■ Consider two important facets of one's reputation; honesty and integrity.

• We tend to indiscriminately lump them together in a kind of moral mush.

- However, speaker and author Stephen Covey,[3] offers some discriminating guidance. He says, "Honesty is telling the truth—in other words conforming words to reality." He goes on to say, "integrity is conforming reality to our words, in other words, keeping promises and fulfilling expectations." Stated differently, honesty is retrospective and integrity is prospective.

- Honesty is what we say about what we've done and integrity is what we do about what we've said.

▫ Old fashioned as the following advice may sound, it is offered with all sincerity: Tell the truth, keep your word, do your share of the work, give credit where credit is due, and don't blame others.

▫ The behavioral expectations of pharmacists are more specific and more demanding than society at large. For example, when working with patients, physicians, pharmaceutical representatives, or contracting agencies through which we receive services, we attain knowledge and information which may be confidential or sensitive. Sharing such information with other clients and other contacts, although it might appear helpful, is blatantly unethical and, therefore, potentially damaging to our reputations. Protecting your reputation within business and professional circles requires a working familiarity with ethics codes established by the pharmacy profession. Pharmacy codes such as the Oath of a Pharmacist[4] endorsed by the American Association of Colleges of Pharmacy (AACP) and the Code of Ethics for pharmacists adopted by the American Pharmaceutical Association (APhA) and endorsed by the American Society of Health System Pharmacists (ASHP) contain strong provisions providing patient and colleague confidentiality and respect. For example, the APhA[5] code states:

    A pharmacist respects the covenantal relationship between the patient and the pharmacist. A pharmacist promotes the good of every patient in a caring, compassionate and confidential manner. A pharmacist acts with honesty and integrity in professional relationships.

▫ A pharmacist respects the values and abilities of colleagues and other health professionals.

- ☐ Good intentions are not enough. Naivete can do you in. Ignorance is no excuse. We should know what is expected within the profession of pharmacy.

- ☐ Years ago, my wife and I purchased a crystal wine decanter as a memento of a visit to Toronto. Each person's reputation is like a handcrafted crystal piece.

  - Like the crystal, each person's reputation is unique.
  - Like the crystal, each person's reputation has many facets.
  - Like the crystal, a long time is required to create a reputation.
  - Like the crystal, once damaged, a reputation may never be repaired.

- ☐ Finally, good news about people travels fast; bad news even faster.

Apply some of the following approaches to personal and professional development

- ☐ Personal and professional development can include developing understanding of and competence in goal setting, personal time management, communication, delegation, personality types, networking, leadership, the socio-political process, and effecting change.

- ☐ Professional development can, in addition to the preceding, include career management, increasing discipline knowledge, understanding business fundamentals, contributing to the profession, and attaining licensure and specialty certification and additional graduate studies.

- ☐ Take charge of your personal development by using these three learning mechanisms available to you as a practicing professional:

  - Just-in-time on the job learning
  - Classes, seminars, and workshops
  - Active involvement in professional societies

- ☐ Enhance the content and accelerate the implementation of your personal and professional development plan by finding a mentor. The mentor should be someone you know and trust and preferably not be your boss. Select someone who will respect confidences and offer constructive criticism and advice. A mentor can be a sounding board and perhaps your safety net.

▣ Holding a current pharmacist license is one indication that you have probably completed the demanding formal education and acquired basic experience. Furthermore, because of ever more demanding licensure laws, licensure indicates that you are maintaining at least minimal competence through continuing education. Pharmaco-therapy board certification, or additional graduate study degrees provide an edge in essentially all areas of pharmacy practice. If you intend to practice pharmacy earning a pharmacy degree and not becoming licensed, board certified, seeking a residency, or attaining continuing education is like buying a sports car and leaving it in the garage.

Consider these ideas on investing for the future

▣ Because of the power of compound interest and the long-term appreciation of stocks, you can build a large retirement fund. Fur-thermore, given the vagaries of the employment market, prudent investing will also quickly accumulate a financial safety net.

▣ However, you must start investing early, and if you haven't started yet, then start now. Avoid this trap: "Wow, that dime of every dollar idea is great! As soon as I can afford it, I'm going to do it."

▣ Project retirement needs and monitor progress toward meeting those needs.

▣ Consider retaining the services of a financial advisor to help you decide how much to invest and how to allocate your investment advisor. A typical annual cost of such services is one percent of the assets managed.

Apply the approaches described elsewhere in this book to enhance communication competence

▣ Depending on your communication strengths and weaknesses,

selectively study the lessons in the "Communication" section of this book. (Note that after the section titled "Personal Roles, Goals and Development," the "Communication" section is the second largest section of this book. And rightly so given the critical role communication ability plays in personal success.)

Consider these thoughts on the importance of networking

▢ Network-network-network, if you are or someday might seek employment. That's essential for all of us. As a pharmacy director, I have conducted numerous personnel searches. We avoided newspaper and similar ads whenever possible because, no matter how tightly written, they attracted too many unqualified candidates which, in turn, required considerable time to process. We focused, instead, on people we knew, knew of, or were referred to us.

▢ One of the best ways to network is to become actively involved in a few, carefully selected professional and community organizations. The emphasis here is on active involvement, rather than passive membership. If you focus on making contributions, contacts will occur and good things will happen. Why? Because you will be known as a competent and contributing individual. People like that make great employees.

▢ Do not join a professional or community organization primarily to make contacts. Your motive will be obvious to most, especially if you contribute little or nothing.

▢ An important aspect of networking and cultivating contacts is carefully choosing your teachers, supervisors, business partners, and colleagues. These associations are especially important early in your career because they deeply influence your attitude about and approach to professional work. Strive to associate with ethical, creative, entrepreneurial individuals.

Read the following related lessons

▢ Lesson 9, "Keeping Our Personal Financial Score"

- ▢ Lessons 12 through 18 in Part 2, "Communication"
- ▢ Lesson 40, "Eagles and Turkeys"

Study the following sources cited in this lesson

1. Goodwin DK. *No Ordinary Time*. New York: Simon & Schuster; 1994.

   Gives a fascinating account of U.S. growth in military and industrial might during World War II, 1994.

2. Handy C. *The Hungry Spirit: Beyond Capitalism: A Quest for Purpose in the Modern World*. New York: Broadway Books; 1998: 61-67.

   Provides an additional, but somewhat negative, discussion of loss of guaranteed employment and the loss of guaranteed employability.

3. Covey SR. *The 7 Habits of Highly Effective People*. New York: Simon & Schuster; 1990.

4. American Association of Colleges of Pharmacy. Oath of a Pharmacist.

   Developed by the American Pharmaceutical Association Academy of Students of Pharmacy/American Association of Colleges of Pharmacy Council of Deans (APhA-ASP/AACP-COD) Task Force on Professionalism; June 26, 1994. Available at: http://accp.org. Accessed July 28, 2007.

5. Proceedings of the 47th annual session of the ASHP House of Delegates. Code of ethics for pharmacists. *Am J Health-Syst Pharm*. 1996; 53:1805.

The psychological contract between employers and employees has changed.
The smart jargon now talks of guaranteeing "employability," not "employment,"
which means ... don't count on us, count on yourself,
but we'll try to help if we can.

— Charles Handy

Afraid of Dying, Or Not Having Lived?

IIIIIIIIIIIIIIIIIIIIIIIIIIIIIIIIIIIIIIIIIIIIIIIIIIIIIIIIIIIIIIIIIIIIIIIIII

We all live under the same sky,
but we don't all have the same horizon.

— Konrad Adenauer

Rabbi Harold S. Kushner, in his book *Living a Life That Matters*,[1] says "The dying have taught me one great lesson...most people are not afraid of dying, they are afraid of not having lived."

We pharmacists have a wealth of resources to help us live full lives; to avoid having "not lived" regrets. Although not the highest, our compensation is certainly adequate. Frankly, we are generally of above-average intelligence, which was one of the reasons we were admitted to pharmacy colleges in the first place. Our education, experience, and caring attitude enables us to define medication-related problems, create treatment plans, compare alternatives, recommend choices, and work with physicians and nurses to implement the desired course of action. Changing employment or finding employment after employment lapses is fairly easy, subject to availability of a position in our specialty in the area we choose to live.

However, referring back to Rabbi Kushner's observation, we pharmacists have some liabilities that could easily lead to late life regrets. We tend to be cautious which, given our responsibilities for patients' safety, health and welfare, is usually an appropriate trait. However, our cautious nature may narrow our vision of what we might do with the rest of our lives. We also tend to be very logical and to rationalize; we are prone to excessive quantification and uncomfortable with ambiguity. For example, in a moment of personal brainstorming, if we were to contemplate dropping out of employment for a year and doing something very different, any one of us could probably come up with ten reasons why we couldn't or shouldn't.

Do not be too timid and squeamish about your actions. All life is an experiment.

— Ralph Waldo Emerson

In the late 1990's, my wife and I decided to move from the familiar surrounds of southeastern Michigan where both of us were raised to the coastal city of Charleston, South Carolina. This was a big change and many of our friends wondered why we would move from the family-oriented community we lived. Many thought we would return within a year or two. As it has turned out, our family and good friends from Michigan visit us often and now easily understand the wisdom of our move. In fact they applaud the fact that we followed our dreams and tell us about some dream or fantasy they had. Based on these and other experiences, I conclude that most of us have visions of unusual things we would like to do. These ideas, if acted on, constitute energetically and creatively living our lives.

Well, let's do at least some of them. Let's avoid entering the golden years with regret for not having fully lived. Hike the Appalachian Trail, open a coffee shop, follow our favorite baseball team on road trips across the country, take flying lessons, join a college faculty, do nothing for a year. Yes, I know there are many reasons why we can't. But there is one overwhelming reason why we should: we only go around once.

Make sure you smell the roses
before you push the daisies.

— Anonymous

Suggestions for Applying Ideas

Grab pen and paper and start a list of things you've repeatedly dreamed of doing, experiences you fantasized about. This might be a joint effort with one or more loved ones or friends.

- ▢ For each item, ask yourself why you want to do it. "Because" is an acceptable default answer.

- ▢ Then, for each item, indicate why you "can't do it" and what you fear.

- ▢ Select one dream or fantasy item; your first choice. View the reasons you "can't do it" and the fears not as barriers but instead as obstacles to be overcome or problems to be solved. Create an action plan to overcome or solve each of them.

- ▢ Start to implement your plan.

Courage is resistance to fear,
mastery of fear,
not absence of fear.

— Mark Twain

Avoid "but-phobia" or "but-neurosis" and, instead, practice the "other side of but."[2, 3]

- ▢ "But-phobia" and "but-neurosis" refer to the tendency to make a positive statement and then immediately follow it with a negative thought leaving, on the balance, a negative, pessimistic message.

- For example: "Traveling in Europe for three months would be a wonderful educational experience, but we could not afford it."

- Or: "Writing a journal article would be satisfying, but I don't have the time."

- Author Marcus Bach, in his book *The World of Serendipity*,[2] advises us to consider "the other side of but." He suggests that "To reverse your point of view is to start your life anew." More specifically, he suggests revisiting the way we say things to make the "but" part of our statements positive.

- Following his advice, the preceding negative statement about European travel could be turned around to become this positive statement: "The 3-month European trip will be educational and expensive, but we will embark on a four-year savings program to generate the necessary funds."

- Or, the defeatist journal article writing expression could be turned around to become this winning expression: "The satisfying article writing experience will require a major time investment, but I will schedule one hour of writing per day for the next 6 weeks to launch the project."

If you think small,
you'll stay small.

— Ray Kroc

Interject the previously mentioned living energetically and creatively idea into your daily and weekly routine. While you can't stop the treadmill, you can hop off for a while. For example:

- Take a different route when you drive or walk home from your office.

- Rent a convertible for your birthday, take a drive in the country with someone special, and have a picnic.

- Stop and browse in that funky gift shop you've passed hundreds of times.

- Enroll in an cooking class.
- Fly to London for a long weekend.
- Send a special card to your spouse, friend, or colleague; just for the heck of it.

Read the following related lessons

- Lesson 7, "Courage: Real and Counterfeit"
- Lesson 8, "Go Out On a Limb"
- Lesson 40, "Eagles and Turkeys"

Study one or more of the following sources cited in this lesson

1. Kushner HS. *Living a Life that Matters.* New York: Knopf, 2001.
2. Bach M. *The World of Serendipity.* Marina Del Ray, CA: DeVorss & Company, 1970.
3. Walther GR. *Power Talking: 50 Ways to Say What You Mean and Get What You Want.* New York: Berkley Books, 1991.

Visit this website

- "Making a Life, Making a Living" (http://www.makingalife.com/) is maintained by Mark A. Albion. As suggested by the title, meaningful living is stressed. This website markets products and includes a free quote search feature.

The mind, ever the willing servant,
will respond to boldness,
for boldness, in effect,
is a command to deliver mental resources.

— Norman Vincent Peale

Part 2

|||||||||||||||||||||||||||||||||||||||||||||||||||||||||||||||||||||

Communication

"The problem was communication." How often have we heard this as the explanation of or excuse for failure or a less than satisfactory result? You missed an important meeting, the poster was printed with the old data, we lost a high performing employee—more often than not, poor communication is the cause; it is not an excuse hiding the real cause.

Communication, or lack thereof, does not have to cause problems; it can prevent them. We can turn communication as a liability into communication as an asset. How? Strengthen our communication knowledge, skills and attitudes and exercise the self-discipline needed to apply them.

Presented in this section are a wide variety of communication ideas and applications intended to elevate awareness of the importance of communication and to enhance your communication competence. Various communication modes are addressed ranging from the all-important asking and listening to preparing, presenting and publishing professional papers.

Lesson 12

Communicating Four Ways

||||||||||||||||||||||||||||||||||||||||||||||||||||||||||||||||||||||||||||||||||||||||||

He who thinketh by the inch
and talketh by the yard
should be kicketh by the foot.

— Walter A. Johnson

To realize our potential in our work, community and personal lives, we must communicate effectively. The most exciting vision, the most thoughtful insight, the most elegant solution and the most creative design are all for naught unless they are effectively communicated to others.

If you lack the ability to communicate well, the intellectual and other seeds that you plant with colleagues, friends, family, and others are not likely to germinate, sprout, and bear fruit, denying others of the bounty of your labors. Communication competence is especially important if we want to develop career security.

With rare exception, effective communication skills are vital to realizing potential and earning career security. Unless you are the non-communicative genius in the work place or the recent graduate who also happens to be the boss's daughter or son, recognition and advancement are dependent on your ability to communicate.

Pharmacists need to know and practice the following four forms of communication:

- ☐ **Visuals:** Visual communication includes the graphics and props used in a presentation as well as the speaker's dress and body language.

- ☐ **Writing:** Pharmacists routinely write emails, memos, letters, chart notes, reports, and other documents. Those of us who want to improve our managing and leading skills should see writing as an essential function that warrants continuous improvement. William Zinsser, a writer, editor and teacher, linked writing and leadership by noting that "Writing is the handmaiden of leadership; Abraham Lincoln and Winston Churchill rode to glory on the back of a strong declarative sentence." Management writer and speaker Thomas L. Brown recognized both the challenge and value of good writing when he said "Hard writing makes for easier reading."

- ☐ **Speaking:** Within pharmacy practice, speaking takes many forms ranging from informal presentations for small groups to formal papers delivered at national conferences. Effective managing and leading requires mastery of this skill. Work on vocabulary, intonation, and accent. Unfortunately, many of us are not comfortable speaking. Journalist Roscoe Drummond, said "The mind is a wonderful thing. It starts working the minute you're born and never stops until you get up to speak in public." None of us can escape speaking, as explained by speaking consultant and author Bert Decker, who said, "...we are all public speakers. There's no such thing as a private speaker—except a person who talks to himself."

- ☐ **Listening:** This easy to overlook communication channel is essential to building interpersonal relationships. When practiced at its best, listening means hearing and understanding words as well as the feelings accompanying them. Stephen Covey, speaker and author, admonishes us to "Seek first to understand, then be understood.[1]" And the Bible (James 1:19) advises us to "be quick to hear, slow to speak, slow to anger."

The complete communicator is competent in all four forms of communication and excellent in some. Through a judicious blend of self-discipline and practice, we can continue to improve our communication ability—and the quality of our lives and those around us.

The difference between the right word and the almost right word is the difference between lightning and the lightning bug.

— Mark Twain

Suggestions for Applying Ideas

Take action to enhance your communication competence

- ◘ Offer to take notes at a meeting—and strengthen your observing, listening, and writing skills.

- ◘ Ask to help present at a staff meeting or interdisciplinary meeting (e.g., nursing inservice) and enhance your speaking and visual skills.

- ◘ Join Toastmasters International (http://www.toastmasters.org/) and develop your own speaking style

- ◘ Volunteer to draft a policy to be implemented either department- or institution-wide.

- ◘ Design a form of education (e.g., flyer explaining standard administration times), which communicates a complex concept or process and appreciate how differently individuals respond based on wording and visual stimuli.

- ◘ Listen to the words for facts, and between the words for feelings, before responding; begin to "hear" what is not said.

- ◘ Examine one of your recently completed projects, identify a portion that would be of interest to your peers, and propose a paper for presentation at a state, regional, or national conference and strengthen your speaking skills and reputation and that of your organization.

Avoid euphemisms, which may amuse, but also confuse[2]

TABLE 12–1. WHAT WE SAY AND WHAT WE PROBABLY MEAN	
WHAT WE SAY	**WHAT WE PROBABLY MEAN**
For your information	I don't know what to do with this, so you keep it
Program	Any assignment that can't be completed in one day
Reliable source	The taxi driver who brought me to work
Give us the benefit of your thinking	We'll listen as long as it doesn't interfere with what we've already decided to do
It is in process	It's so wrapped up in red tape the situation is probably hopeless

Recognize differences between the way women and men communicate in the workplace[3]

TABLE 12–2. COMMUNICATION TENDENCIES IN WOMEN AND MEN	
WOMEN TEND TO:	**MEN TEND TO:**
Use disclaimers: "This may be a silly question, but…"	Be assertive: "It is obvious that…"; "Note that…"
Foresee a crisis, head it off, don't make it a big deal.	Allow a crisis to happen, solve it, and take the credit for the good deed.
Be indirect: "The billing clerk needs help. What would you think of helping her out?"	Be direct: He would tell the employee to help the billing clerk.
Give way to a male's interruption, let him take over.	Interrupt, then talk over the person he interrupted.
Listen with eye contact, frequently nodding, indicating understanding and approval.	Listen with stoic expressions, eyes off in another direction, revealing nothing.
Pause, waiting for indications of approval or understanding, and allowing others to contribute.	Speak in a steady stream without pauses. Not allowing others to join the conversation.

TABLE 12–2. COMMUNICATION TENDENCIES IN WOMEN AND MEN (CONT'D)	
WOMEN TEND TO:	**MEN TEND TO:**
Solicit opinions before stating a position, to make others feel involved.	State viewpoint unequivocally, and take on challengers.
Say "we."	Say "I."

Determine the possible influence of body language on some of your recent positive and negative experiences

If the words were "right on" but the desired effect did not occur, your body language may not have been aligned with the intended message.[4-6]

- ▣ A combination of smiling, relaxed posture and unrestrained movement suggests happiness or satisfaction.
- ▣ Frowning, tense posture, and a rigid body or nervous movement indicates unhappiness or dissatisfaction.
- ▣ Nodding, winking, smiling and relaxation usually suggest agreement.
- ▣ Side-to-side head movement combined with frowning and crossed arms project disagreement.

Communication is not what is intended,
but what is received by others.

— Mel Hensey

Recognize, both as a receiver and an initiator, the four principal types of communication flow in all types of organizations[7]

- ▣ *Downward*, or enabling, communication that moves instructions and other directive information down or through a hierarchy.
- ▣ *Upward*, or compliance, communication that provides feedback to the people who originate downward communication.

- *Lateral*, or coordinating, communication that moves between peers to maintain or improve operational efficiency.

- The *grapevine*, which fills in gaps in official communication and provides answers to unaddressed questions.

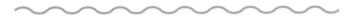

Mental telepathy is not, I fear,

a reliable means of communicating in most organizations.

— Charles Handy

Read the following related lessons

- Lesson 10, "Job Security is an Oxymoron, Career Security Doesn't Have to Be."

- Lessons 12 through 18 (Part 2, "Communication")

Study one or more of the following sources cited in this lesson

1. Covey SR. The 7 *Habits of Highly Effective People: Restoring the Character Ethic*. New York: Simon & Schuster; 1990.

2. Loeffelbein B. Euphemisms at work. *The Rotarian*. 1992;(Feb):22–23.

3. Tannen D. *Talking from 9 to 5: How Women's and Men's Conversational Styles Affect Who Gets Heard, Who Gets Credit and What Gets Done at Work*. (audio cassette) New York: Simon and Schuster Audio, 1997.

4. Hendricks M. More than words. *Entrepreneur*. 1995;(Aug):54–57.

5. National Institute of Business Management. *Body Language For Business Success*. New York: NIBM; 1988.

6. Reinhold BB. Body language. *U.S. Airways Magazine*. 1997;(March):8–13.

7. Abbott RF. "Downward communication: enabling communication," (Sep. 1); "Upward communication: compliance," (Sep 8); "Lateral communication: coordination," (Sep 22); and The grapevine: defying the rules," (Sep 29). *Abbott's Communication Letter*. 1999.

Study one or more of the following supplemental sources

▣ Benton DA. *Lions Don't Need to Roar: Using Leadership Power of Professional Presence to Stand Out, Fit In and Move Ahead.* New York: Warner Books; 1992.

Offers tips on speaking, listening and visual messages.

▣ Cialdini RB. The science of persuasion. *Scientific American.* 2001;(Feb):76–81.

Contends that "six basic tendencies of human response come into play in generating a positive response" to a request. They are reciprocation, consistency, social validation, liking, authority, and scarcity.

Subscribe to one or more of these e-newsletters

▣ "Abbott's Communication Letter," a free monthly e-newsletter produced by Robert F. Abbott. Included are practical ideas, presented in an anecdote format, you can use everyday to help you and your organization succeed. To subscribe, go to http://www.abbottletter.com/.

▣ "Qmail," a free questioning oriented e-newsletter available from Organization Technologies, Inc. To subscribe, contact dleeds@dorothy.leeds.com.

In order to speak short on any subject, think long.

— Hugh Henry Brackenridge

Lesson 13

So What Do You Know About Macaws?

||||||||||||||||||||||||||||||||||||||||||||||||||||||||||||||||||||||||||||||||||||||||||

I had six honest serving men—they taught me all I knew:
their names were Where and What and When—
and Why and How and Who.

— Rudyard Kipling

When our son was in high school, he invited me and my wife to the school's annual recognition banquet. Dinner would be followed by presentations and entertainment. Upon arriving, our son saw a friend who was there with his parents. After introductions, the six of us sat down for dinner.

Initially, there was little conversation. To break the awkward silence, I abruptly asked the group, "So, what do you know about macaws?" This question, which came out of the blue, simultaneously embarrassed my son and drew some smiles. It broke the ice and we enjoyed a pleasant conversation. (My motivation for asking the question was really to learn about macaws, or more specifically, severe macaws. We were in the process of buying one from a breeder.)

My son frequently kids me about the "embarrassing" macaw question of years ago. Recalling the incident, along with considerable subsequent experience taught me the benefits of questions. One benefit is that it enables mildly introverted individuals (like me) to engage people in conversations in social settings. Most people will answer almost any positive question you ask them and, quite frankly, seem to enjoy the attention.

In a conversation, keep in mind that
you're more interested in what you have to say
than anyone else.

— Andy Rooney

Asking questions has also helped me throughout my career. On the surface, success as a healthcare leader might seem to be a function of what you know. In actual practice, however, success is closely linked with how effectively you learn what you need to know. Much of the knowledge you need is acquired by asking many questions of the stakeholders. Some questions uncover facts and others reveal feelings.

Asking the right questions
takes as much skill as
giving the right answers.

— Robert Half

As pharmacists, the quality of our service is a function of what we know about those we serve, their environment and their needs. We gain that knowledge by asking thoughtful, open-ended questions intended to stimulate informative answers. More bluntly, we don't learn much when we do all the talking. Maybe that's why we have one mouth, two ears, and two eyes. Maybe that's why "So, what do you know about macaws?" suggests a powerful means of building personal and business relations.

The most important thing in communication is to hear what isn't being said.

— Peter Drucker

Suggestions for Applying Ideas

Consider the seven powers of questions[1]

1. Questions demand answers.
2. Questions stimulate thinking.
3. Questions reveal valuable data and information.
4. Questions put the questioner in control.
5. Questions encourage people to open up.
6. Questions lead to quality listening.
7. Questions cause people to persuade themselves.

Improve your questioning ability by applying some of the following tips

- Arrange to meet and ask questions of the right people. Try to talk with knowledgeable people who have decision-making authority.
- Prepare for a conversation by listing questions you would like to ask.
- Strive to achieve the 20/80 rule; you making statements and asking questions no more than 20% of the time and listening at least 80% of the time.
- Minimize focus on you—limit use of "I," "me," "we," "our," …
- Maximize focus on them—generously use "you," "your," …
- Mix close-ended and open-ended questions. Close-ended questions are typically answered with yes, no, or a statement of fact. In contrast, open-ended questions lead to thinking, expressing of opinion, and discussion.

◻ Start open-ended questions with active verbs like explain, clarify, analyze, and translate.

◻ Strive for empathetic listening, that is, acquire information and understand feelings.

◻ Listen for emphasis and respond accordingly. The following is a statement made to a pharmaceutical representative. Note the four varied meanings of the following sentence based on which words are emphasized:

- *I* don't think, at this time, we would be interested in purchasing your product.

- I don't think, *at this time*, we would be interested in purchasing your product.

- I don't think, at this time, *we* would be interested in purchasing your product.

- I don't think, at this time, we would be interested in *your product*.

◻ Ask questions of strangers.

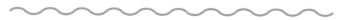

Children ask better questions than adults.

— Fran Lebowitz

Recognize the five levels of attentiveness (listed from most to least attentive)[2,3]

1. Empathetic listening: hearing everything plus understanding feelings (most attentive).

2. Attentive listening: hearing everything.

3. Selective listening: hearing only what we want to hear.

4. Pretending to listen: hearing nothing but looking like we do.

5. Ignoring: hearing nothing and looking like we hear nothing.

Verify your understanding of what is being said

- ▢ Occasionally saying, "I see," "tell me more!" or similar.
- ▢ Maintaining eye contact.
- ▢ Not interrupting.
- ▢ Exhibiting positive, receptive body language.
- ▢ Paraphrasing.
- ▢ Sketching or drawing.
- ▢ Asking additional clarifying questions.

Read the following related lessons

- ▢ Lesson 14, "Talk to Strangers"
- ▢ Lesson 39, "Interviewing So Who You Get Is Who You Want"

Study one or more of the following sources cited in this lesson

1. Leeds D. *The 7 Powers of Questions: Secrets to Successful Communication in Life and Work.* New York: Perigee, 2000.
2. Covey SR. *The 7 Habits of Highly Effective People.* New York: Simon & Schuster; 1990.
3. Decker B. *You've Got to Be Believed to Be Heard.* New York: St. Martins Press; 1992.

Refer to the following supplemental source

- ▢ Hensey M. *Personal Success Strategies: Developing Your Potential.* Reston, VA: ASCE Press, 1999.

    Chapter 12 presents a "what I know chart" that can be used to stimulate question asking. The four levels of knowing outlined in the chart are (1) know that I know; (2) know that I don't know; (3) think I know, but don't; and (4) don't know that I don't know.

~~~~~~~~~~~~~~~~~~~~~~~~~~~

*Nature, which gave us two eyes to see and two ears to hear,
has given us but one tongue to speak.*

— Jonathan Swift

Subscribe to this e-newsletter

▫ "Qmail," a free questioning oriented e-newsletter available from Organization Technologies, Inc. To subscribe, contact dleeds@dorothyleeds.com

~~~~~~~~~~~~~~~~~~~~~~~~~~~

Let every man be quick to hear,

slow to speak,

slow to anger.

— James 1:19 Bible, *Revised Standard Version*

Talk to Strangers

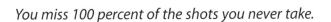

You miss 100 percent of the shots you never take.

— Wayne Gretzky

The advice suggested by the title of this lesson contradicts what our parents told us to do when we were children. However, we are no longer children and presumably can take care of ourselves. In her book, *How to Work a Room*, consultant Susan RoAne challenges her readers to "work the world."[1] She urges us to adopt the philosophy that we are surrounded by opportunities to learn and make contacts. But we often have to take the initiative, whether we are at our place of work, doing personal errands in our community, sitting in an airport between flights or attending a conference.

Will talking to strangers always yield useful information or a new contact? Certainly not. However, RoAne says:

> That's not the point. The point is to extend yourself to people, be open to whatever comes your way, and have a good time in the process. One never knows … The rewards go to the risk-takers, those who are willing to put their egos on the line and reach out—to other people and to a richer and fuller life for themselves.

Writing this lesson caused me to contemplate some positive results of conversations I've had with strangers. For example, I:

- ☐ received an appointment to a high-level professional commission partly as a result of introducing myself to a society staff member and suggesting that we share conversation and a cab ride to the airport.

- ☐ found an effective personal time management system as a result of talking to a stranger on an airplane. I learned that he conducted time management seminars and he gave me a sample of the system he used.

- ☐ identified a strong candidate for a pharmacy informatics position as a result of introducing myself to a person I did not know at the opening reception of a state society meeting.

Talking to strangers can be a challenge. It might be difficult to know what to talk about. Frankly, most people like to talk about themselves and their interests. Therefore, give them an opportunity to do so by asking questions. If they are half as thoughtful as you are, they will reciprocate and many pleasant and informative conversations will result. Even if they don't reciprocate, you'll probably learn something by asking sincere questions. The person who asks questions, directs the conversation and benefits the most from it.

If you enjoy a conversation you had with a person you've met, that's a good reason to take action. Exchange business cards. A thoughtful follow up might be as simple as an email or handwritten note to them saying, "It was a pleasure meeting you. I enjoyed our conversation. I hope to see you in the future."

Each lifetime is the pieces of a jigsaw puzzle.
For some, there are more pieces.
For others, the puzzle is more difficult to assemble.
But know this:
You do not have within yourself all the pieces to your puzzle.

Everyone carries with them at least one
and probably many pieces to someone else's puzzle.

— Lawrence Kushner

Suggestions for Applying Ideas

Prepare yourself to start a conversation the next time you enter a reception, icebreaker, or similar event[2]

- ⬚ Adopt this mindset: I am here to meet, learn, help, and possibly start mutually beneficial relationships.

- ⬚ Wear your nametag.

- ⬚ Have a supply of quality business cards handy.

- ⬚ Seek out strangers; not only but mostly.

- ⬚ Prepare a ten second description of what you do, sometimes called an "elevator speech." Mine is: "I manage pharmacy services within a health system."

- ⬚ Keep moving—five to ten minutes per person or small group will work.

- ⬚ Ask for a business card as you meet or are about to leave someone. If they asked you for something or you made a promise, note it on their card.

- ⬚ Listen 80 percent of the time; talk and ask 20 percent. As soon as possible after the event, fulfill all promises and make other follow-ups as appropriate.

Ask open-ended questions (i.e., questions that cannot be answered "yes" or "no") when you want to encourage conversation but can't think of a way to start

- ⬚ "What do you hope to get out of this meeting?"

- ⬚ "I notice that you work in home infusion services—what attracted you to that area of pharmacy?"

◻ "I am working on a medication safety-related project and need some ideas. Does anybody in your organization do this?"

◻ "I have never been to your part of the country. What is it like to live there?"

Consider these thoughts on serendipity when you hesitate to start a conversation[3]

◻ Serendipity may be defined as the process by which we "dip" into life with "serenity."

◻ Serendipity means "catching on to the magic of the thing called chance;" of "making discoveries by accident ... of things not in quest of."

◻ While we may have a particular goal in mind in talking to strangers, we may serendipitously achieve some other benefit.

Record the essentials of what you learn as strangers become contacts, and sometimes colleagues or even friends

◻ Even if you don't aggressively follow the "talk to strangers" advice of this lesson, you will in the course of your work and other activities, meet hundreds, if not thousands of individuals.

◻ Experience clearly indicates that you will have need to contact many of these individuals for various reasons such as data, information, referrals, collaborative projects, and employment. A contact could occur months, or even years, after meeting a person.

◻ Useful data and information to note about a contact include name, employer, title and credentials, address, telephone and fax numbers, email address, special interests, and names of spouses, children, and mutual acquaintances.

◻ Use some form of electronic system, such as your email directory, to record data and information about members of your growing network.

You can make more friends in two months
by becoming really interested in other people,
than you can in two years
by trying to get other people interested in you.

— Dale Carnegie

Read the following related lessons

- Lesson 6, "DWYSYWD"
- Lesson 8, "Go Out On a Limb"
- Lesson 13, "So What Do You Know About Macaws?"

Study one or more of the following sources cited in this lesson

1. RoAne S. *How to Work a Room: A Guide to Successfully Managing the Mingling.* New York: Shapolsky Publishers; 1988.

2. Entreprenuer.com 2002. "Power-schmoozing your way to the top"; (May 6) 2002. http://www.entrepreneur.com/marketing/marketingideas/networking/article51570.html

3. Bach M. *The World of Serendipity.* Marina Del Rey, CA: DeVorss & Company; 1970.

Refer to one or more of the following supplemental sources:

- Benton DA. *Lions Don't Need to Roar: Using the Leadership Power of Professional Presence to Stand Out, Fit In, and Move Ahead.* New York: Warner Books; 1992.

  Stresses the need to match professional competence with the ability to make personal connections. Offers advice on physical appearance, greeting strangers, gestures, listening and voice variation.

- Leeds D. *The 7 Powers of Questions.* New York: Perigee; 2000.

  Claims that questions demand answers, stimulate thinking, reveal data and information, control the conversation, encourage others to speak, enhance listening, and persuade.

Subscribe to this e-newsletter

◫ "Qmail," a free questioning oriented e-newsletter available from Organizational Technologies, Inc. To subscribe, contact info dleeds@dorothy.leeds.com.

No matter how ambitious, capable, clear-thinking, competent, decisive, dependable, educated, energetic, responsible, serious, shrewd, sophisticated, wise, and witty you are, if you don't relate well to other people, you won't make it. No matter how professionally competent, financially adept, and physically solid you are, without an understanding of human nature, a genuine interest in the people around you, and the ability to establish personal bonds with them, you are severely limited in what you can achieve.

— Debra A. Benton

Balance High Tech and High Touch

||||||||||||||||||||||||||||||||||||||||||||||||||||||||||||||||||||||||||||||||||||||

All of the technology in the world will not help us
if we are not able, at the core,
to communicate with each other
and build strong, lasting relationships.

— Dorothy Leeds

Today's electronic communication and data gathering devices are amazing. Many of us frequently, often daily, use voicemail, teleconferencing, fax, email, pagers, PDAs, and the worldwide web. The next wave of widely used electronic communication devices is already appearing and includes more wireless tools; live, multi-station audio-video conferencing; "smart" documents; and individualized, self-paced, web-based education and training. And who knows what is beyond that.

We derive numerous and varied business and professional benefits from this electronic "wizardry." For example, it enables us to quickly and cost-effectively:

■ Send and receive valuable patient information with various members of the healthcare team.

- Function as virtual teams and benefit from collaboration even though we may work in scattered locations
- Work on national committees within our professional organizations
- Conduct research using global resources
- Manage multi-health-system projects and programs
- Recruit personnel and market services

There is a potential downside, however. Over reliance on electronic communication technology can actually reduce interpersonal communication. We can lose meaningful contact with our colleagues, fellow healthcare practitioners, patients, regulators, citizens, and stakeholders.

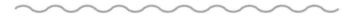

… our practice must be based on the basic belief that Pharmacy is ultimately not about technology, computers, budgets, or even drugs but about people we serve and our genuine love respect, and concern for them.

— Billy W. Woodward

The literature reveals few studies evaluating personality traits of pharmacists. With regard to communication, these studies suggest a slightly noticeable degree of introversion and avoidance of interpersonal communication.[1] Stated differently, excessive use of electronic devices can push us even closer to the introvert end of the introvert-extrovert spectrum, and as a result, take us further from meaningful, empathetic (facts plus feelings) interaction with others. As busy, multi-tasking professionals, we may be tempted to say that when I can communicate electronically, rather than personally, I will. After all, if some electronic communication is good, isn't more better?

Success in the pharmacy profession is ultimately based on the trust each of us earns from our stakeholders. Earning and maintaining trust requires some meaningful human interaction, that is, "face time," "eyeball-to-eyeball" conversation, and empathetic listening. Communication that is efficient, that uses the latest electronic devices, is not necessarily effective especially when it becomes the only mode of interaction.

Let's frequently and skillfully use electronic tools but intersperse that use with human interaction. Electronic devices are tools used in communication, they are not communication. Let's balance their high tech with our high touch.

Technology does not improve the quality of life;
it improves the quality of things.
Improving the quality of life
requires the application of wisdom.

— Neil Armstrong

Suggestions for Applying Ideas

Personalize the communication between yourself and others

◻ Before establishing another committee or project team, get the members together for a "kick-off" working and social event. Create an opportunity for them to become acquainted and to connect. This may encourage more face-to-face communication in the future.

◻ As you begin to compose the "umpteenth" email, pick-up the telephone instead and suggest that the two of you meet face-to-face or "do lunch."

◻ Rather than sending a generic thank you email or memorandum to the members of your team for a job well done, compose a personalized, handwritten note to each person and send it via "snail mail" or, better yet, hand it to them with a brief statement of appreciation.

Read the following related lessons

- ▣ Lesson 12, "Communication: Five Ways"
- ▣ Lesson 28, "TEAM: Together Everyone Achieves More"
- ▣ Lesson 29, "Virtual Teams"

Study the source cited in this lesson

1. Nimmo CM, Holland RW. Transitions in pharmacy practice, part 4: Can a leopard change its spots? *Am J Health-Syst Pharm.* 1999;56:2458–2462.

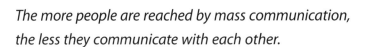

The more people are reached by mass communication, the less they communicate with each other.

— Marya Mannes

Trimming Our Hedges

|||||||||||||||||||||||||||||||||||||||||||||||||||||||||||||||||||||||||||||||||||||||||||||

On speaking,
first have something to say,
second say it,
third stop when you have said it.

— John Shaw Billings

Pharmacists are, by and large, decent individuals. They want to be open and honest in their interactions with others. That desire, taken to extremes, leads to over explanation of results that others may perceive as lack of competence, confidence, or commitment

What is needed is some "hedge-trimming": the ability to speak, write, and answer questions in a positive manner, to present our views without excessive qualifications, so that the information is presented at the level of appropriate for our intended audience.

For example, at a staff meeting, do not answer a question about the required procedure for medication reconciliation with "If I read the policy correctly..." We are responsible for understanding policies correctly, and communicating the correct procedures to employees. In contrast, a qualified answer such as "based on the limited data, in my opinion there will be no problems" would be an acceptable qualification in responding to questions from professional peers who understand the complexity of our work.

As another example, that same statement ("Based on limited field data...") would not be appropriate to present to a public body. The "in my opinion" part of the statement is sufficient.

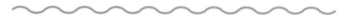

Mastery of language affords remarkable power.

— Frantz Fanon

What we say and how we say it influences others' opinions of us, our work, and the organizations we represent. The tendency to over-qualify statements and responses suggests the following negatives to listeners: inadequate preparation, lack of ability, low self-confidence, or insensitivity to colleagues. These perceived traits can detract significantly from the image and performance of the professional. Left uncorrected, this could interfere with advancement within the organization and the profession. More importantly, these negative impressions can frustrate the implementation of viable recommendations. The fact that we are well prepared, have ability, are confident and competent is irrelevant if we are perceived to be otherwise. Perception is fact.

We should do all assignments well. When explaining or reporting the results to others, we must be very sensitive to the nature and interest of the audience. Let's speak in simple, declarative, and brief fashion unencumbered with excessive, convoluted qualifications.

Incidentally, the preceding focuses on how what we say influences others. What we say and how we say it also influences ourselves. Consider the more positive effect on your subsequent performance when you say, "I will get the draft report to you by Friday noon" rather than "I will try to get the report to you by Friday noon." Less hedging leads to more personal commitment. Let's trim our hedges.

The ancestor of every action
is a thought.

— Ralph Waldo Emerson

Suggestions for Applying Ideas

Listen for hedges in your communication

Table 16–1 illustrates how the words we use in routine conversation set high or low expectations for ourselves and those around us.[1-3]

Study the following sources cited in this lesson

1. Hill N. *Think and Grow Rich.* New York: Fawcett Crest; 1960.

2. Roger J, McWilliams P. *Do It! Let's Get Off Our Buts.* Los Angeles, CA: Prelude Press; 1991.

3. Walther, G. *Power Talking: 50 Ways to Say What You Mean and Get What You Want.* New York: Berkley Books; 1991.

For one word a man is often deemed to be wise,
and for one word he is often deemed to be foolish.
We should be very careful indeed what we say.

— Confucius

TABLE 16–1. HOW WORDS SET EXPECTATIONS

Indicates Low Expectations	Indicates High Expectations
I'll have to …	I'll be glad to …
I'll try to …	I will …
I can't do …	I haven't done … but want to learn how
This is a problem	This is an opportunity
I will spend on education and training	I will invest in education and training
This is impossible	This is going to require a special effort
Excuse my messy office	Welcome to my place
I've just been here one month but maybe …	I've observed the situation since starting a month ago and suggest …
I got lucky	I set goals and acted constructively to achieve them
I performed poorly	I learned …
If only I …	I will …
She just doesn't understand …	I will try another way to explain …
That's your problem …	Let's try …
This should take a few weeks …	I will get it to you by …
To tell the truth …	(Just tell it)
You don't remember me …	Good to see you again, my name is …

P⁵: *Preparing, Presenting, and Publishing Professional Papers*

Pharmacy leaders or pharmacists who are seeking to become leaders, should search for opportunities to present posters at meetings or publish research and other information in professional journals

— Sara J. White

Preparing, presenting, and publishing professional papers (P⁵) is a concrete means of giving something back to the pharmacy profession. P⁵ also provides the following personal and organizational benefits:

- Improved writing and speaking ability which is directly and immediately transferable to many aspects of our professional and personal lives.
- Increased confidence as a result of interacting with peers.
- Expanded visibility of our organization with emphasis on its accomplishments and abilities.
- Earned membership in networks of leaders which provides quick access to assistance when needed.

Presenting and publishing may sound like a great idea with clearly evident benefits—a win-win-win-win all around for the audience, the profession, your employer, and you. But you probably think you don't have the time to prepare, present, and publish a paper. In actuality, the extra investment in time and effort to produce a paper typically will be very small compared to the substantial effort you and others have already expended on a potential paper's subject. The following paragraphs describe and thereby simplify the P^5 process.

Content. You do not need to first do special work that would serve as the subject for a paper. Instead, you and potential co-authors should seek to write papers about the good work that you are doing or already have done. Aspects of current projects, which may seem routine to you because of your immersion in them, may be exciting and valuable to your peers. Scan your current or recently completed projects for potential topics.

Of course, you may be doing work the results of which are not worth sharing with the profession. If all or most of your efforts are producing such marginal results, are you practicing sound stewardship with your education, experience, and potential? If not, perhaps you should lead internal changes or move on to an employer whose work is worth speaking and writing about.

Getting on the Program. With your topic in hand, seek possible conferences for presentation of your as-of-now unwritten paper. Learn about upcoming conferences by noting published calls for papers, reading articles in professional society periodicals, skimming flyers announcing conferences, visiting websites of professional organizations, and using your network.

Having identified one or more appropriate conferences, write and submit an abstract of your still unwritten paper. Theoretically, the abstract should be written after the paper is drafted. Realistically, the abstract is usually written before the paper is written. This backward approach works well provided you already have, as a result of your project involvement, the material you will need and you have thought through the structure of the presentation, at least in a conceptual fashion.

Writing the Paper. Assuming your abstract is accepted, immediately begin to outline and write the paper. Do so even if a written paper is not a condition for oral presentation at the conference. The three benefits of developing a written paper are:

1. Having exercised the discipline and applied the thought required to prepare a written paper, we are **better prepared** for the oral presentation.

2. The written paper can be provided, electronically or in hardcopy, prior to, or after the presentation, to anyone who requests it or to individuals we think might be interested. This use of the written version **expands the paper's audience and influence,** strengthens our personal network, and enhances the reputation of our organization.

3. Having the written paper available facilitates the usually desirable last step in the P⁵ process; **publication** in a journal or periodical.

Presenting the Paper. As the presentation time approaches, don't assume anything. Verify audio-visual equipment. Check out the presentation room at least 1 hour before your presentation or the start of the session containing your presentation. Prepare a short written biographical sketch which the host or session chair could use to introduce you. Speak directly to the audience; not to the screen, your notes, or the ceiling. The audience is not there. Prompt questions, answer those you can, and to follow up on the others.

The courage to speak
must always be balanced
by the wisdom to listen.

— Benjamin Franklin

Publishing the Paper. Some conferences produce proceedings, that is, a collection of written versions of the presented papers. Having one's paper in the proceedings helps to extend its longevity, expand its availability, and leverage its influence.

If a proceedings is not produced, the organization sponsoring the workshop is likely to publish journals or other periodicals. Determine which of these is most appropriate and obtain the paper submittal requirements. Revise the written paper to comply with those requirements and to reflect input received during and after the oral presentation. If the sponsoring organization does not produce journals or other periodicals, find an appropriate professional organization that does and work with them.

Suggestions for Applying Ideas

Look for potential topics for papers among your current or recently completed projects

- ☐ A new technology or a new application of an existing technology.
- ☐ An innovative process to more effectively involve pharmacists in direct patient-care activities.
- ☐ A procedure for conducting benefit-cost analyses on budget requests.
- ☐ An unusual means of funding a research and/or performance improvement project.

Structure your overall presentation around T³

- ☐ Tell them what you are going to tell them.
- ☐ Tell them.
- ☐ Tell them what you told them.

Ask yourself what you would like members of the audience to do as a result of hearing you

- ☐ Some possible answers:
  - Try an interdisciplinary approach that you found useful.
  - Take at least one step toward developing more leadership ability.
  - Advocate a change in the standard of practice.

- Use your department's services.

▫ Align all aspects of your presentation with the desired action or actions of your audience. That is, as you determine what to say and how to say it, consider what you want audience members to do.

▫ Explicitly tell your audience what you hope they will consider doing as a result of your presentation. This should be an integral part of the T³ mentioned previously.

~~~~~~~~~~~~~~~~~

A speech without a specific purpose is like a journey without a destination.

— Ralph C. Smedley

Recognize and prepare for the different preferred learning and understanding styles that are likely to be present in your audience

▫ Basic learning styles are:

- Auditory: understand mainly by hearing
- Visual: understand principally by seeing
- Kinesthetic: understand mainly by touching and doing

▫ Prepare for the visually-oriented members of your audience by using photographs, line drawings, graphs, cartoons, icons, and videos.

▫ Interact more effectively with the visual learners by selecting colors to symbolize or convey messages. Some possible examples are listed below:[1]

Blue	trust, authority, security
Green	money, growth, environment
Orange	movement, construction, energy
Pink	femininity, calm
Purple	royalty, spirituality
Red	power, activity, rescue
Yellow	light, future, philosophy

▫ Communicate with the visual and kinesthetic-oriented participants by using props such as an example of a particular medication administration device, a model, or a demonstration.

Leverage your published paper or article

▫ Send copies to individuals who participated in or contributed to the work in the paper thanking them for their help.

▫ Insert copies, as appropriate, in your annual employee performance evaluation and in your department or institution's annual report.

▫ Use your organization's website or newsletter to advise others of the availability of the paper.

▫ Prepare variations on the paper, possibly including new developments or emphasizing other aspects, and use the revised paper as the basis for a new presentation-publication cycle.

Read the following related lessons

▫ Lesson 18, "Practice Out Loud"

▫ Lesson 43, "Giving to Our Profession and Our Community"

Study the following source cited in this lesson

1. Raskin A. The color of cool. *Business 2.0.* 2002;(Nov): 49–52.

Refer to the following supplemental resource

▫ Carnegie D. *Public Speaking and Influencing Men in Business.* New York: Association Press; 1948.

Although old, as is evident from the use of the word "men" in the title, this book offers many ideas to help you prepare for and deliver a speech. The underlying message is that there is no "silver bullet" for becoming an effective speaker; adopt sound principles and practice, practice, practice.

I love being a writer.
What I can't stand is the paperwork.

— Peter De Vries

Lesson 18

Practice Out Loud

||||||||||||||||||||||||||||||||||||||||||||||||||||||||||||||||||||||||||||||||

Practice is the best of all instructors.

— Publilius Syrus

Pharmacists have numerous opportunities to make, or help to make, presentations. Typical audiences are colleagues within our organizations, other healthcare practitioners such as physicians and nurses, members of professional associations, service clubs, patients, and students. The professional and business community places a high premium on the ability to make effective presentations. Individuals who develop good to excellent speaking skills are well-regarded as measured by span of influence, promotions, compensation, perquisites, added opportunities, and perhaps most important of all, personal satisfaction for a difficult task well done.

One of the most powerful ways to prepare for delivering an effective presentation, once the all-important content is in hand and organized, is to practice it out loud. Practicing out loud means exactly that. It does not mean "saying" the words to yourself.

Practice your presentation out loud, including use of visuals and props, preferably in front of one or more people with whom you feel comfortable and who are likely to offer constructive criticism. If you are not able or inclined to do that, practice your presentation out loud in the privacy of your office, home, hotel room, the room in which you will make the presentation, or some other location. Never give a presentation without having practiced it out loud several times, even if only to yourself. Equally important, never memorize a presentation. An audience will immediately detect memorization and will cease to listen attentively.

Three reasons are offered for out loud practice:

1. Out loud practice **establishes the actual time** required to give a presentation. Reading or speaking the presentation to ourselves makes us likely to greatly underestimate the delivery time. Most presenters are given a specific time allotment. If you underestimate the time required to deliver your talk, you risk going over and, in turn, agitating the audience, offending other speakers, and embarrassing yourself and your organization.

If I am to speak ten minutes,
I will need a week's preparation.
If 15 minutes, three days.
If half an hour, two days.
If an hour, I am ready now.

— Woodrow Wilson

2. Each time we practice a presentation "out loud," we **become more knowledgeable** about the content of our speech. We discover additional words and phrases to say what we want to say. We master words that were initially difficult to pronounce. We discover aspects of our topic that require further investigation or elaboration. When we actually make our presentation to the audience, we will, accordingly, have more experience to draw on. We will already have given a similar speech several times. Many good speeches that have been well prepared in terms of content and organization, are spoiled

because the speaker seems to be searching for the right words. Although, this probably reflects the lack of out loud practice, not a lack of substantive content or familiarity with material. However, the audience is likely to perceive the latter.

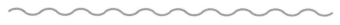

How can I tell what I think till I see what I say?

— Edward Morgan Forster

3.　Practicing a presentation out loud to trusted colleagues or to family members helps us ***identify and reduce distracting habits***. Playing with change or keys in our pockets, interspersing hedges such as "ah" and "you know," avoiding eye contact, looking at just a portion of the audience, and speaking to the screen instead of the audience – all are examples of distractions. Others are mispronouncing words, speaking in a monotone, using unusually long sentences, rocking back and forth, and frequently taking off and putting on glasses.

Another way to practice is to speak frequently on a variety of topics in a variety of settings to a variety of audiences. If each time we speak, we receive critiques and audience feedback, we will become more effective speakers.

Good to great speakers, like good to great actors, athletes, and musicians, make it look easy and we as listeners and viewers benefit. Experience suggests, however, that what looks easy is the result of hard work, one aspect of which is out loud practice.

Suggestions for Applying Ideas

Make an audio recording, or better yet, an audio-video recording, of your practice session

▣　This is especially useful if you are reluctant to practice your presentation out loud with a live audience or are unable to do so.

▫ A simple way to record the audio for at least a portion of your presentation is to call your home or office telephone number and leave a voicemail that is all or a portion of your out loud practice. What you hear may not sound the way you think it does.

▫ A video recording offers the added benefit of enabling you to see how you say what you say. Body language is an essential element. Assume, for example, that you inadvertently and often cross your arms across your chest while speaking. Many audience members will interpret this as a signal that your mind is made up and that you are not open to other perspectives or options, even though your words say otherwise. What you say and how you appear when you say it should be aligned.

Experiment with techniques you admired in accomplished speakers

▫ Technique examples include gestures, props, alliteration, unusual visuals, varying volume and pace, and moving into and out of the audience.

▫ Study effective speakers, in person, on television or on videotapes. Note the techniques that work for them.

▫ View each of your presentations as an opportunity to experiment with at least one new approach. Try mimicking some of the techniques you've seen and heard other speaker's use, with suitable modifications for your personality and the particular presentation. Your goal is developing more effective means of communication.

Experience the real sound of your voice

▫ Unless you have listened to and studied a recording of your voice, you do not know the real sound of your voice. You are likely to be surprised!

▫ According to speaking consultant and author, Bert Decker[1], "…the voice on the tape is much closer to what others actually hear than the voice we ourselves hear as we speak." The voice we hear when we speak is conducted largely through the bones in our head while the voice others hear is transmitted through the air. Decker notes that the "reel" voice is the "real" voice, at least as far as your audiences are concerned.

☐ Unless you plan to talk only to yourself, you ought to know how you sound to others. If you don't like it, change it.

☐ Record all or part of your next presentation as part of your preparation to speak. A small micro-cassette recording device that you turned on and unobtrusively placed on the lectern or otherwise near you at the beginning of your talk will capture the verbal and vocal components of your presentation. Privately study the recording, identify strengths and weaknesses, and explicitly build on the former while you diminish the latter.

We are all public speakers.
There's no such thing as a private speaker—
except a person who talks to himself.

— Bert Decker

Memorize a few, selected portions of your presentation

☐ The opening statement—to create a strong beginning.

☐ The closing statement—to assure that the intended message has been communicated and to transition to questions and discussion.

☐ Quotations—to ensure you repeat them correctly.

Visualize your complete presentation and the audience's response

☐ Assemble a profile of the likely audience by conferring with organizers of the event, visiting the sponsoring organization's website, and using your network. Learn enough about the audience so that you can approach them from their perspective. Include items such as the following in the audience profile:

- Likely number

- Disciplines/specialties represented

- Education

- Age

- Years of practice/work

- Gender

- Reasons to be present

▫ Based on the audience profile, identify one or more ways to connect with all or portions of the audience near the beginning of your presentation. Perhaps you share a professional discipline, have worked on or are working on similar projects, or have lived in their geographic area.

▫ Learn what you can about the room or space within which the presentation will occur. If feasible, visit the room well before the actual presentation to learn first hand about it and possibly practice your presentation out loud. Items of interest include audience-seating arrangements (e.g., classroom, U-shaped), presence of a stage or platform, location of the screen relative to the audience, and availability of a remote control if you are using PowerPoint or a similar graphics system.

▫ With information like the preceding in hand, practice your presentation out loud again this time visualizing where you will be relative to the audience and what you will be doing to enliven communication.

▫ Practice moving about the room, making gestures, changing voice cadence and volume, pausing, using props, and speaking directly to particular members of the audience, other speakers, and the moderator. Wear the type of clothing you are likely to wear when you actually speak.

▫ In a sense, the entire room is your stage—at least while you are speaking. You are the producer, director and actor. Use visualization to fully utilize all verbal, vocal, and visual communication channels.

~~~~~~~~~~~~~~~~~~~~~~~~~

Practice does not make perfect.
Only perfect practice makes perfect.

— Vince Lombardi

Ask a spouse, family member, friend or colleague to attend your actual presentation and provide you with a frank critique

- Encourage them to watch and listen to you while observing the audience. Ask them to listen to what audience members say among themselves during and after your presentation. Request that they record audience questions.
- What were your strengths?
- What needs improvement?
- Commit to building on your strengths and making improvements.

Read the following related lesson

- Lesson 17, "P⁵: Preparing, Presenting, and Publishing Professional Papers."

Study the following source cited in this lesson

1. Decker B, Denney J. *You've Got to Be Believed to Be Heard.* New York: St. Martin's Press; 1992.

Refer to the following supplemental source

- Urban H. *Life's Greatest Lessons: 20 Things That Matter.* New York: Simon & Schuster; 2003.

  Chapter 11, "Real Motivation Comes from Within," urges us to create mental pictures of the success we desire, noting that we don't think in words; we think in pictures.

Subscribe to one or more of these e-newsletters

- "Abbott's Communication Letter" is a free monthly speaking tips e-newsletter from Robert F. Abbott. To subscribe, go to http://www.abbottletter.com.

- "Great Speaking" is a free speaking tips e-newsletter produced by Advanced Public Speaking Institute. To subscribe, go to http://www.public-speaking.org.

- "The Professional Speaker" is a free weekly e-newsletter that offers speaking tips. Example topics are use of humor, caring for the audience, and telling stories. To subscribe, go to http://www.professionalspeaker.com.

Visit one or more of these websites

- "Advanced Public Speaking Institute" (http://www.public-speaking.org) is the website of the *Advanced Public Speaking Institute*. Available free speaking resources include checklists (e.g., a detailed pre-program questionnaire), a large public speaking glossary, and over 100 articles and links to other websites.

- "National Speakers Association" (http://www.nsaspeaker.org/) is maintained by the NSA. This organization "provides resources and education to advance the skills, integrity and value of its members and the speaking profession." Included on the website are information on joining the organization, coming events, and a free knowledge bank and resource center that you can search using key words or phrases.

- Presentation Skills, Public Speaking, Professional Speaking (http://www.antion.com) is the website of Antion and Associates. Very commercial with numerous materials and items for sale. Also offers free articles.

- "Toastmasters International" (http://www.toastmasters.org/) is the website of Toastmaster's International, which has the tagline "making effective oral communication a worldwide reality." Included are free speaking tips, access to an online store offering a wide variety of products, and information on how to find a Toastmaster's International Club near you.

The notes I handle no better than many pianists.
But the pauses between the notes—
ah, that's where the art resides.

— Arthur Schnabel

Part 3

||||||||||||||||||||||||||||||||||||||||||||||||||||||||||||||||

Learning and Teaching

Ideally, each of us would, on a daily basis, learn and teach. Most of us have the ability to do both. All of us have the responsibility to do the latter, in the spirit of helping others by sharing what we know, and the need to do the former. Success in a science and technology-based profession like pharmacy on each individual's and each organization's ability to keep up with new developments. In addition, we share with all professions the need to study and understand changing social, economic, environmental, and political conditions.

This section offers suggestions for individual learning, one-on-one learning and teaching, and group efforts. The underlying theme: our responsibilities as manager and leaders include learning and teaching.

Lesson 19

Garage Sale Wisdom

||||||||||||||||||||||||||||||||||||||||||||||||||||||||||||||||||||||||||||||||||||||||

The man who does not need good books
has no advantage over the man who can't read them.

— Mark Twain

My wife enjoys garage sales and, although much less enthused, I often go with her. Upon arrival, she typically traverses all the treasures while I head for the inevitable piles or boxes of old books. Our roles reverse in used bookstores, I enjoy cruising the stacks and my wife is a good sport by coming along.

Books at garage sales and in used bookstores cover the waterfront ranging from those labeled "Two years or younger" to encyclopedia sets that end with World War II; from romance novels to medical reference books. My targets tend to be biographies, histories, and management and leadership books. As a result of visits to garage sales and used bookstores, I have found some interesting books all of which, although secondary, were terrific bargains.

A garage sale yielded Napoleon Hill's *Think and Grow Rich*[1] published in 1960. I had heard of, but never read, this enlightening book. Contrary to the narrow monetary theme suggested by the title, Hill explains how he searched for the secret that enabled a few individuals to achieve great significance and success, financial and otherwise. The secret, based on Hill's 25-year study, is the power of visualization and the subconscious mind.

Management and Leadership,[2] authored by Carl F. Braun, president of a manufacturing firm, was purchased for a nickel at a Florida garage sale. Consider some thoughts from this book: "A company cannot rise above its people." Teamwork occurs when the leader practices "teaching, helping, guiding, encouraging" in contrast with using "decree, dictate, command." "Ethics is not a trimming to the business tree. It is a mighty root of it." "Few leaders fully grasp the meaning of the verb, to lead,…to initiate,…to instruct and guide,…to take responsibility, …to be out in front." This book, which offers advice consistent with today's most enlightened thinking, was published in 1954!

Harper's Anthology for College Courses in Composition and Literature—Prose,[3] was purchased in the used book section of a Florida shop. Included in this 1926 book are the maxims of the French moralist Francois La Rochefoucald. One example of his 17th century thoughts applicable to today is "As it is the characteristic of great wits to convey a great deal in a few words, so, on the contrary, small wits have the gift of speaking much and saying nothing." And consider the appropriateness of this thought for pharmacists and the crucial nature of our judgment: "To know things well, we should know them in their details; but as their details are almost infinite, our knowledge is always superficial and imperfect."

Other garage sale/old bookstore volumes in my library include:

- ▪ Dale Carnegie's *Public Speaking and Influencing Men In Business,*[4] first published in 1926 and purchased at an Indiana garage sale,
- ▪ *The Human Side of Enterprise,*[5] published in 1960 by Douglas McGregor and found in a New Jersey used bookstore, and
- ▪ *Essays*[6] by Ralph Waldo Emerson, published in 1936 and found in a Florida shop.
- ▪ *The Deming Management Method*[7] published in 1986 by Mary Walton and found at a South Carolina garage sale.

Buying old books has benefited me in two ways. First, I have acquired useful skills and knowledge by reading the books; my knowledge and perspective have been expanded. For example, Napoleon Hill's *Think and Grow Rich* discovery fleshed out some of my earlier intuitive thinking. Second, given that the books mentioned in this essay were all originally published two or more decades ago and offer observations and advice similar to that offered today, I am gradually concluding that those things that are really important change little over decades, if not centuries.

They say what goes around comes around. Garage sale and similar older books in my library suggest a possible variation on the preceding; the tried and true, while they may be ignored, never go away. Reading old books helps distinguish the truly new from the superficial, the wheat from the chaff.

I keep to old books,
for they teach me something;
from the new I learn very little.

— Voltaire

Suggestions for Applying Ideas

Purchase some "garage sale wisdom," skim it or read it, and consider the following questions

▣ What's different between then and now both with regard to the book's subject matter and about the social, economic, and political environment?

▣ Are the differences matters of substance or of minor significance?

▣ What new ideas and information did you find in the old book?

Take a new look at some of your old college books and other books

▣   This suggestion assumes that you are somewhat like me in that you have difficulty getting rid of old books. Perhaps your old books have a place of honor in your office or den, or maybe they are stored, and almost forgotten in the attic, basement or garage.

▣   What do these "old friends" have to say today in contrast with your recall from back then? Some possibilities:

- You now have an answer for some of those question marks you placed on various pages.

- An idea you read about back then in one of your liberal arts courses proved to be a turning point for you; it profoundly influenced the direction of your life.

- You realize that, although you thought you knew much back then, you didn't. You still don't know much relative to what you now understand about what there is to know.

Book: A garden carried in a pocket.

— Arabian proverb

Read the following related lesson

▣   Lesson 20, "Read and You Won't Need a Management Consultant"

Study the following sources cited in this lesson

1. Hill N. *Think and Grow Rich.* New York: Fawcett Crest Book Company; 1960.

2. Braun CF. *Management and Leadership.* Alhambra, CA: C.F. Braun & Company; 1954.

3. Manchester FA, Giese WF, eds. *Harper's Anthology for College Courses in Composition and Literature.* New York: Harper and Brothers, 1926.

4. Carnegie D. *Public Speaking and Influencing Men In Business.* New

York: International Committee of the Young Men's Christian Associations; 1948.

5. McGregor D. *The Human Side of Enterprise.* New York: McGraw-Hill; 1960.

6. Emerson RW. *Essays.* Reading, PA: The Spencer Press; 1936.

7. Walton M. *The Deming Management Method.* New York, NY: Perigee, 1986.

*To add a library to a house
is to give that house a soul.*

— Marcus Tullius Cicero

Lesson 20

Read and You Won't Need a Management Consultant

A man is known by the company his mind keeps.

— Thomas Bailey Aldrich

President Harry S Truman once said, "There is nothing new in the world except the history you do not know." In keeping with the spirit of his statement, I doubt that there are many employee, department, or organizational problems within the pharmacy profession that haven't occurred and been solved before.

After reflecting on my pharmacy experiences, I conclude that few pharmacists read about management, leadership and related topics. This strikes me as unfortunate for them, because the literature is rich with ideas and information on how each of us can assess our skills, articulate our aspirations, and create and implement a personal improvement action plan.

Not all readers become leaders.
But all leaders must be readers.

— Harry S Truman

Are you inclined to read more widely in and beyond the management and leadership area? If so, I respectfully suggest that you consider some of the following:

▢ *7 Habits of Highly Effective People*[1] by Stephen Covey. Unlike many of the gimmicky self-help books, Covey's focuses on application of sound personal and interpersonal principles to achieve win-win outcomes.

▢ Jim Collin's *Good to Great: Why Some Companies Make the Leap...and Others Don't.*[2] This book discusses the common traits that 11 successful companies possess and ways to make those traits work for your organization.

▢ Donald McHugh's *Golf and the Game of Leadership.*[3] Starting on the "practice tee" and taking you through 18 "holes," the book defines the basic principles to golf and leadership.

▢ *Working with Emotional Intelligence* [4] by Daniel Goleman. Goleman discusses emotional intelligence as a set of five crucial skills that sets stars apart from the mediocre and shows how they determine our success within relationships and work.

▢ *First, Break All the Rules: What the World's Greatest Managers Do Differently*[5] by Marcus Buckingham and Curt Coffman. The authors outline four factors to become an outstanding manager: finding the right fit for employees, focusing on strengths of employees, defining the right results, and selecting staff for talent.

▢ *The 21 Indispensable Qualities of a Leader: Becoming the Person Others Will Want to Follow*[6] by John Maxwell. Maxwell's chapters are titled by "character qualities" that includes character, charisma, commitment, communication, competence, courage, discernment, focus, generosity, initiative, listening, passion, positive attitude, problem-solving, relationships, responsibility, security, self-discipline, servant hood, teachabililty, and vision. Within each chapter he provides anecdotes and exercises for personal improvement to each of the character qualities.

▢ *Manager's Toolkit: The 13 Skills Managers Need to Succeed*[7] by The Harvard Business School Press. This book is focused on the needs of new managers to provide guidance, coaching, and tools on topics such as hiring, budgeting, and setting goals.

◫ Stuart Levine's *The Six Fundamentals of Success: The Rules for Getting It Right for Yourself and Your Organization.*[8] Practical book on the six fundamentals that include: add value, communicate well, deliver results, act with integrity, invest in relationships, and gain perspective.

Never attribute to malice

what can be explained by incompetence

because incompetence really is

so much more common that deliberate malice.

— Josef Martin

The answers to your personal, project, and organizational managing and leading challenges are "out there." One way to obtain those answers is to read deeply and broadly.

Suggestions for Applying Ideas

Follow Mortimer Adler's advice on "how to read a book"[9]

◫ Take an active role in your reading. For example, as you read, frequently answer this question in your own words" "What is really being said?" Then consider questions like "Is it true?" and, if so, "How can I use it?"

◫ Take notes, perhaps in the book's margins. Include ideas, information, questions, and action items.

◫ Test yourself. That is, as a result of reading the book what new ideas and information did you acquire and, more importantly, how will your thinking and behavior change as a result?

~~~~~~~~~~~~~~~~~~~

He that reads and grows no wiser
seldom suspects his own deficiency,
but complains of hard words and
obscure sentences, and asks why
books are written which cannot be
understood.

— Samuel Johnson

Read widely and eclectically

◻ Many of the readings suggested in the lesson are not explicitly connected to managing and leading.

◻ This implies the power of eclectic reading, that is, occasionally reading books, periodicals, newspapers and other materials drawn from outside of our normal reading patterns and not necessarily related to our work. Consider reading biography, history and phi-losophy. Eclectic reading also means reading articles and books with points of view different than yours.

◻ We can also eclectically view television, listen to the radio, and attend the theater. However, the advantage of eclectic reading is that we can stop and ponder what we read; we control the pace.

◻ If you don't normally do so, occasionally read newspapers such as the *New York Times* and the *Wall Street Journal,* and magazines and other periodicals such as *Fortune, Harvard Business Review, Modern Healthcare,* and *Money.*

◻ Eclectic reading may provide a fresh perspective on tried and true processes, offer a glimpse of future technologies and service needs, expand your vocabulary, provide added insight into human nature, and introduce you to new opportunities.

All things are filled full of signs,

and it is a wise man

who can learn about one thing from another.

— Plotinus

Read the following related lesson

- Lesson 19, "Garage Sale Wisdom"

Study one or more of the following sources cited in this lesson

1. Covey S. *The 7 Habits of Highly Effective People.* New York: Simon & Schuster; 1990.

2. Collins J. *Good to Great: Why Some Companies Make the Leap...and Others Don't.* New York: Harper Business Press; 2001.

3. McHugh D. *Golf and the Game of Leadership.* New York: AMACOM; 2004.

4. Goleman D. *Working with Emotional Intelligence.* New York: Bantam Books; 1998.

5. Buckingham M, Coffman C. *First Break All the Rules: What the World's Greatest Managers Do Differently.* New York: Simon & Schuster; 1999.

6. Maxwell JC. *The 21 Indispensable Qualities of a Leader: Becoming the Person Others Will Want to Follow.* New York: Nelson Business Press; 1999.

7. Harvard Business School Press. *Manager's Toolkit: The 13 Skills Managers Need to Succeed.* Harvard Business School Press; 2004.

8. Levine SL. *The Six Fundamentals of Success: The Rules for Getting It Right for Yourself and Your Organization.* New York: Doubleday; 2004.

9. The essence of Mortimer Adler's 1940 book *How to Read a Book* is summarized in R. Grugal. 2002. Reading is an art form. *Investors Business Daily.* May 5.

Reading maketh a full man,
conference a ready man,
and writing an exact man.

— Francis Bacon

Caring Isn't Coddling

||||||||||||||||||||||||||||||||||||||||||||||||||||||||||||||||||||||||||||||||||||||||||

It's a funny thing about life;

if you refuse to accept anything but the best,

you very often get it.

— W. Somerset Maugham

In my role as residency program director, I recall a meeting with one of the postgraduate year two (PGY 2) residents who had a challenging personal situation. The resident's dog that she loved very much was expected to pass away within the next few days. She had come to me to request to be excused from attending the regional residency conference where she would present her residency project because she wanted to be with her dog through his last few days. After a few moments of thought, my response was that she did not need to attend the conference but would need to present her project at a future pharmacy staff meeting. I found this decision difficult, but did decide on the basis of what I thought was important to this person at this time in her personal life.

As we develop our personal relationships, in the department, within pharmacy organizations, and in the pharmacy profession, many of us hope that a strong element of caring will be evident in our actions toward others and in their actions toward us. Caring, as used here, does not mean coddling. Well then, if caring isn't coddling, what is it?

To answer this, think about those former elementary, high school, or college professors who really cared about you. They probably demonstrated their concern for you narrowly as a student and broadly as a person through a variety of meaningful interactions. Examples are: delivering well-prepared lectures, making regular and demanding assignments intended to deepen and broaden understanding of the course material, providing opportunities for independent study such as a research paper or laboratory project, encouraging you to participate in extra-curricular leadership and professional organization service activities, offering an encouraging word at a discouraging time, and praising when nobody else seemed to notice what you had accomplished.

The preceding were not offered in a paternalistic, condescending, ostentatious manner; rather these actions were part of high expectations—high support environment intended to stretch without snapping, provide example without expecting cloning, and build confidence without imparting arrogance.

Give the other person a
fine reputation to live up to.

— Dale Carnegie

Caring is also exemplified by the parent who says, "if its worth doing, its worth doing well" and the colleague who, at a meeting, has the courage to ask the awkward question or raise the sensitive issue that almost everyone knows must be addressed. Caring is also shown by the manager who says no to the pleading employee who did not strive to meet the established requirements and now wants to avoid the adverse consequences.

You may also recall, with disdain, those professors, supervisors, colleagues, and others who were generally "nice" but didn't expect all that much of you. Often times you delivered in accordance with their expectations. You and they could have done so much more. Perhaps they didn't really care about you, or even themselves.

Caring isn't coddling. Caring is pushing, pulling, admonishing, stretching, demanding, encouraging, urging, challenging, cajoling. Caring is high expectations coupled with high support. Caring helps individuals and organizations meet their goals and realize their full potential.

What is honored in a country
will be cultivated there.

— Plato

Suggestions for Applying Ideas

Recall someone who, during a formative period in your life, consistently had high expectations for you and matched those expectations with high support

◘ How did they communicate their expectations?

◘ How did they offer support?

◘ How did you benefit?

◘ What did you learn from that relationship that might enable you to, in turn, offer high expectations—high support to others?

The nature of our discipline is the sum
total of the inner drives – that is, the souls –
of individual practitioners.

— William A. Zellmer

Pass along the benefits of high expectations—high support

◘ Select someone you oversee who would benefit from structured guidance.

◘ Initiate the kind of high expectations—high support experience that enriched your life.

◫ Articulate your and/or your department's expectations for the selected person.

◫ Pledge your and the department's support if the employee strives to meet the stated expectations or some mutually agreeable variations.

◫ Hold the selected person accountable to develop as expected and hold yourself and your department accountable to provide support as warranted.

◫ After a few months, reflect on the success of your efforts. Did your supervisee benefit from your coaching like you benefited from the efforts of your coach or mentor?

Read the following related lessons

◫ Lesson 2, "Roles, Then Goals"

◫ Lesson 3, "Smart Goals"

◫ Lesson 27, "Delegation: Why Put Off Until Tomorrow What Someone Else Can Do Today"

◫ Lesson 38, "Our Most Important Asset"

Time and money spent in helping men
do more for themselves
is far better than mere giving.

— Henry Ford

More Coaching, Less Osmosis

*The only irreplaceable capital an organization possesses
is the knowledge and ability of its people.
The productivity of that capital depends on
how effectively people share their competence
with those who can use it.*

— Andrew Carnegie

Being a Director of Pharmacy Services has provided me with an opportunity to objectively see vertical slices of various organizations—from entry-level pharmacists and pharmacy technicians on up through middle and senior managers to the CEO or other administrator positions. Experienced leaders within pharmacy typically possess a wealth of knowledge. That is one of the reasons they are where they are. Their knowledge and skills are broad and deep.

Sometimes seasoned managers complain about the ineptness of the more junior manager. These new leaders are, according to the senior personnel, poor communicators, can't manage projects efficiently, get bogged down in clinical matters, and have little business sense.

Unfortunately, the seasoned leaders often have little if any explicit involvement in sharing what they know. Frequently, inexperienced managers are not even told about their non-clinical shortcomings, their management and leadership deficiencies. A common attitude is that an entry-level managers will realize, apparently through osmosis, that they have "soft-side" skill deficiencies and, also by osmosis, learn how to resolve those deficiencies. Osmosis is an effective physical process but not an effective people process.

Most new practitioners within organizations hunger, or should hunger, for knowledge about professional practice, especially the non-clinical or "soft-side" aspects. Some eventually learn, sometimes positively by osmosis, but often negatively through mistakes that are costly and painful for them, their employers, and the organization.

Fortunately, there are several effective ways to leverage the experience of an organization's principals and other upper echelon personnel. Coaching is one of the most effective and efficient approaches. Coaching means occasional, one-on-one focused interactions between an interested senior leader and a receptive junior manager. Senior and junior usually refer to age but could also refer to differences in experience level between two individuals. For example, a new practitioner may have more experience in a specific clinical area then an interested senior person. Accordingly, the new practitioner could coach the more experienced person.

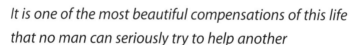

It is one of the most beautiful compensations of this life that no man can seriously try to help another without helping himself.

— Ralph Waldo Emerson

Coaching is distinguished from mentoring which typically requires a major, personal, on-going effort over an extended period—a year or more. Coaching is accomplished intermittently during the course of on-going projects and activities. It is not a separate training activity.

So how can experienced leaders coach others? How will the senior leader have time to fit this additional activity into already busy schedules? The answer is to look, in the normal course of work, for specific coaching opportunities that will take the receptive, junior manager up the "soft-side" skills learning curve and will provide him or her with some management and leadership insights. Tailor the coaching situations to the level, needs, and receptivity of the new manager.

New practitioners are usually quite bright but they don't always know what they don't know, especially if it is outside of the clinical or technical or "hard" side arena. They need to be told, by word and by example, that a judicious blend of clinical and "soft-side" abilities is essential to personal and organizational success. Coaching is a highly leveraged way of sharing management and leadership skills and knowledge. Experience indicates that there can be a terrific return on this investment in the pharmacy profession.

Suggestions for Applying Ideas

Look for an opportunity to coach someone in your organization

- In your role as project manager, invite a inexperienced pharmacist to attend the meeting and observe the proceedings. On the way to the meeting, describe what appear to be the key issues, how they were determined and how they will be discussed. Outline the hoped for outcome of the meeting. After the meeting, jointly and constructively discuss the meeting and critique the tactics and skills of the various participants.

- Work with a student/resident/new practitioner in reviewing a departmental performance report in order to understand the budgeting process, the expenses associated with running the department and how revenue is calculated.[1]

- Provide an opportunity for a pharmacist to participate in interdisciplinary collaboration allowing him or her to develop an understanding of nursing as a customer and the best ways to communicate with nursing to accomplish an organization's project.[1]

☒ Engage the employee in managerial decisions such as staffing needs, interviewing and selecting candidates for employment, performance reviews, and addressing staff termination and complaints. [1]

☒ Invite the new practitioner to participate in the review/revision of documents or lead a meeting that addresses topics such as developing a business plan, policy and procedures, and a staffing schedule. [1]

A coach is someone who can give correction without causing resentment.

— John Wooden

Recognize that some people who do things very well, like public speaking or negotiating, don't know how they do it. Take action to learn from these individuals.[2]

☒ Accept that they cannot explain what they do and, therefore, they are not effective as active coaches. However, such high performers can serve as passive coaches.

☒ How? Arrange for yourself and others to observe those who do things well while they are doing it. Encourage the observers to identify the knowledge, skills and attitudes that explain the admirable performance.

☒ Go one step further, "interview" the exceptional performers as a means of learning more about how they do it. While active coaching may not be their forte, responding to questions may be.

Investigate mentoring, either as an informal effort or as a department program, if coaching proves successful in developing personnel

☒ Mentoring requires much more effort than coaching but, if done well, yields much greater benefits.

☒ Some definitions of mentoring:

• Someone helping someone else learn something the learner

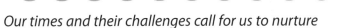

would otherwise have learned less well, more slowly, or not at all.[3]

- One person invests time, know-how, and effort in enhancing another person's growth, knowledge, and skills, to prepare the individual for greater productivity or achievement.[4]

- A labor of love that requires self-denial, courage, time, and altruism. [5]

■ Caution: A department mentoring program requires a major time commitment. Allow at least a year for a trusting and productive relationship to develop between a mentor and the mentee. Many hours of quality time consisting of mentor-mentee conversations and between conversation efforts will be needed during that year.

Our times and their challenges call for us to nurture idealists, who will generate the ideals so desperately needed by our profession as it navigates the future's turbulent seas.

— Henri R. Manasse, Jr.

Read the following related lessons

■ Lesson 38, "Our Most Important Asset"

■ Lesson 40, "Eagles and Turkeys"

Study one or more of the following sources cited in this lesson

1. American Society of Health-System Pharmacists. Helpful Residency/ Rotation/ Internship Ideas for Activities to Provide Leadership Training. http://www.ashp.org/s_ashp/docs/files/ ResidencyLeadershipTraining.pdf. Accessed July 14, 2007.

2. Hensey M. "Core Competencies for Living" (Chapter 5) and "Learning How To Learn" (Chapter 6) in *Personal Success Strategies.* Reston, VA: ASCE Press; 1999.

3. Adapted from Bell CR. *Managers as Mentors*. San Francisco, CA: Koehler Publishers; 1996.

4. Adapted from Shea GF. *Mentoring: Helping Employees Reach Their Full Potential*. AMA Management Briefing. New York: American Management Association; 1994.

5. Pierpaoli P. Mentoring. *Am J Hosp Pharm*. 1992;49:2175–2178.

Visit this website

■ ASHP Virtual Mentoring Exchange (http://www.ashp.org/s_ashp/doc1c.asp?CID=1242&DID=7133). Enrolling in the ASHP Virtual Mentoring Exchange allows both students/new practitioners the opportunity to be teamed up with seasoned pharmacy professional from around the country to provide career related advice via the internet forum.

He has a right to criticize
who has a heart to help.

— Abraham Lincoln

Lesson 23

I Ain't No Role Model

‖‖

"Having a role model in life is a great thing to have;
one who provides us with direction and inspiration.
However, we will forever be restricted by that person's
limitations if we live within their boundaries.
Be influenced, but set your own standards
and develop your own principles."

— Jason Shahan

As a pharmacy professional it is important to remember that "actions speak louder than words," and our practice and behaviors truly do impact the perception of up and coming pharmacy professionals. Another example of professionals who, whether they mean to or not, greatly impact our children and our young pharmacy students and pharmacists, are professional athletes. However, while being interviewed, a "star" athlete once proclaimed "I ain't no role model." Based on their actions, apparently many "professional" athletes share this perspective.

Having observed the way impressionable children watch, idolize, and mimic these athletes, I am concerned about the adverse effect of the "I ain't no role model" approach. Most regrettable are the lost opportunities to teach hard work, self-discipline, fair play, and other positive behaviors.

A visit, several years ago, to the Michael Jordan exhibit at the Chicago Museum of Science and Industry reminded me of the tremendous effort required to achieve excellence in athletics. This valuable lesson is largely missing in today's sports world.

*I never thought a role
model should be negative.*

— Michael Jordan

What a shame, because understanding the cost of high achievement, even for the naturally intellectual or physically gifted, is a lesson that is transferable to many of life's endeavors. And our children and other young people should learn that lesson.

Let's bring this "I ain't no role model" topic closer to home. Consider an example which many pharmacists may relate to. You may have had a similar experience in pharmacy school, such as this one. Imagine attending a pharmacy conference, during which a pharmacy professor participated in a panel discussing the roles of a pharmacy professor and their relationship with students. The pharmacy professor stands up and emphatically states that his responsibilities do not include being a role model for his students. How would you feel? I frankly, having helped precept pharmacy students, and having taught pharmacy classes as an adjunct professor, would be very angry. As a professor, and a mentor, I try very hard to relay the messages of professionalism, ethics, studious behaviors, honesty, and other characteristics that are favorable in a pharmacist.

One or two generations ago, the "do as I say not as I do" modus operandi might have worked with pharmacy students. Not today. In our information-rich society coupled with our highly-inquisitive, headline-seeking press, today's compliance with the well-known proverb provides a steady stream of disconnects between what politicians, business executives, clergy, and academics say and actually do.

Young people see the disconnect. The most enlightened among them will listen respectfully to what you or I say and then carefully watch what we do. They naturally want to know if we are "for real" or our pronouncements are just hot air that they can ignore. Leadership writer John C. Maxwell stressed the importance of what we do relative to what we say this way: "What people need is not a motto to say but a model to see."

Are our actions aligned with, or in conflict with, our words? Are we positive role models? If "yes," then we will constructively influence our students, employees, and colleagues. If our actions are not aligned with our words, we damage our credibility, eventually irreparably, and fail those who want to look up to us, for their good and that of our organization. Ask yourself, do you set the example?

Consider the following examples of when you may need to ensure your actions and behaviors align with those you expect of others:

- If an executive were to call for ethical behavior, are your decisions and actions above reproach?

- As a faculty member, you require timely submittal of assignments, do you start and end your classes on time and honor your posted office hours?

- As a pharmacist lobbying for passing of legislation in your favor, do you advocate meaningful interaction with stakeholders, and routinely and effectively communicate with citizens and other interested individuals?

- As a faculty member, do you stress the need to be open to new ideas, and, at times, lead change? Can you describe situations in which you have worked for and more importantly, led fundamental change?

- As a practitioner or academic, your organization most likely has a published vision and detailed strategic plan. Can you point to your specific, significant contributions to achieving that vision?

We must remember that everyone, especially younger people, are watching. Whether we like it or not, we are role models. The ultimate question is, what are we modeling? Are our words and actions aligned?

The final test of a leader is
he leaves behind him in other
men the conviction and will
to carry on.

— Walter Lippman

Suggestions for Applying Ideas

Read the following related lessons

- ◻ Lesson 1, "Leading, Managing, and Producing"
- ◻ Lesson 2, "Roles, then Goals"
- ◻ Lesson 18, "Practice Out Loud"
- ◻ Lesson 22, "More Coaching, Less Osmosis"

Study one or more of the following supplemental sources

- ◻ Zoller K, Preston K. *You Did What? The Biggest Mistakes Professionals Make.* 3rd ed. Arlington, TX: Tapestry Press. 2002.

  Provides a guide to professionals on setting the example and how to comply with business etiquette.

- ◻ Wollenburg KG. Leadership with conscience, compassion, and commitment. *Am J Health-Syst. Pharm.* 2004: 61:1785–91.

  Discusses the importance in possessing the traits of conscience, compassion, and commitment in the profession of pharmacy and how to possess these traits to lead and be a role model for employee development.

- ◻ Buerki RA, Vottero LD. Ethics for pharmacists. In: Brown TR, ed. *Handbook of Institutional Pharmacy Practice.* Bethesda, MD: ASHP; 2006: 509–518.

  Provides insightful information on how to handle potentially ethical and moral dilemmas which face pharmacists in an institutional pharmacy setting, and how we should represent our profession according to the Code of Ethics for Pharmacists approved by the American Pharmaceutical Association on October 27, 2004

- Chisolm MA, Pritchard L. Influence of pharmacists as role models. *Am J Health-Syst Pharm.* 1995;52(12):1348. Documents and describes the influence of pharmacy practitioners as role models for students that pursued a career in pharmacy.

Visit one or more of these websites

- Josephson Institute of Ethics. http://www.josephsoninstitute.org/business-ethics_links.html This link leads to a list of organizations, colleges, and some solicitations for providing ethics training courses. However, it is a good resource to many websites which focus on professional ethical behavior.
- Character Counts! www.charactercounts.org. Maintained by the Josephson Institute of Ethics. The website contains links to helpful resources and presentations on ethics, and the six pillars of character, primarily for students and children.

The power of one man or one woman
doing the right thing for the right reason,
and at the right time,
is the greatest influence in our society.

— Jack Kemp

Lesson 24

Education and Training: From Ad Hoc to Bottom Line

||||||||||||||||||||||||||||||||||||||||||||||||||||||||||||||||||||||||||||||||

In times of change, learners inherit the earth,
while the learned are beautifully equipped
to deal with a world that no longer exists.

— Roland Barth

Patients increasingly demand services that meet their needs. Serving patients, the organization, and department requires practitioners to have current knowledge and skills in both clinical and non-clinical areas.

A major portion of a hospital or health-system is the knowledge that the employees possess. This is intellectual capital. We are increasingly in the knowledge business. Accordingly, as stated by Benjamin Franklin, scientist, statesman, diplomat, and author, "an investment in knowledge pays the best interest."

Based on the preceding, maintaining and building intellectual assets are essential for the long-term viability of hospitals and health-systems. Pharmacy departments, for example, are increasingly challenged by the constant initiation of new medications into the market, a challenge that may lead to improvement if personnel receive education and training (E&T).

As a result, during the past decade, many pharmacy departments have developed E&T programs to better educate pharmacists and technicians in reviewing the basics of medication management and to also enhance there knowledge of new medications and diseases states. They have shifted from an ad hoc, individually-focused model to a planned, department-focused model.

There are two likely negative reactions to the need to create more structured and organizationally-focused E&T programs. First, a E&T program would "cost too much" and, second, employees will participate in the E&T and then leave taking the investment with them. With respect to the first objection, experience indicates otherwise. Instead of spending more money, the intent is to leverage current expenditures more wisely. In thinking about the second objection, experience also indicates otherwise as suggested by this thought: The only thing worse than educating and training people and having them leave, is not educating and training them and having them stay.

Suggestions for Applying Ideas

Determine which of these nine potential benefits of an organizationally-focused E&T program could be applicable to your pharmacy department[1]

- Articulate and share the organization's culture, that is, its history, values, mission, and goals.

- Attract and retain even higher quality personnel. A dominant characteristic of top-flight personnel is their desire for continuous learning.

- Achieve more effective use of monetary and time resources currently being expended on E&T. This may be accomplished by focusing on the organization's needs (not individual "wants"), using many and varied delivery mechanisms tailored to the learning situation, reducing duplication of efforts, and holding individuals accountable for sharing and/or using what they know.

- Close skill gaps, that is, shrink the differences between what personnel know and what they need to know, or know better, in order to achieve the organization's mission, vision and goals.

◻ Facilitate advancement of individuals, and the commensurate satisfaction and other rewards, by improving knowledge and skills.

◻ Grant continuing education units (CEU's), thus further recognizing employees; assisting them in meeting license, registration, and renewal criteria; and enhancing the stature of the organization.

◻ Improve individual and department productivity and project fiscal performance, leading to improved savings and profitability.

◻ Enhance quality as indicated primarily by meeting the patients and organizations needs and other project requirements.

◻ Hold E&T efforts to specific performance outcomes, at least in the first year or so of operation. The thinking here is that one way to "sell" organizational managers and leaders on a new approach to E&T is to produce concrete supporting outcomes data.

Why, then, do companies manage it [human capital]
so haphazardly?
A principal reason, I believe,
is that they have a hard time distinguishing between
the cost of paying people
and the value of investing in them.

— Thomas A. Stewart

Find the optimum mix of sources and delivery mechanisms for providing E&T lessons, modules, and experiences

◻ While in-house workshops and seminars are likely to be one form of teaching and learning, other potential content sources and delivery mechanisms are:

• Carefully selected books, papers, and articles studied as part of one's personal professional plan, read as pre-module attendance assignments or used as the basis for discussion groups.

- Audio and audiovisual cassettes used individually or in a group setting.
- Computer-assisted, nonlinear, interactive, individualized learning.
- Web-based interactive, individual and group distance learning (synchronous and asynchronous).
- Correspondence courses.
- Conference calling such as sessions at which experts on the topic exchange "tips."
- E-mailing sharing, that is, a mechanism for announcing knowledge and information needs, on the assumption that someone will be able to help, and sharing knowledge and information, on the assumption that someone else may be interested.
- Attendance at external workshops, seminars and conferences sponsored by professional organizations with the expectation to "share" knowledge (e.g., staff meeting presentation) upon return to the office.
- Brown bag presentation of knowledge gained "on the job" or at a workshop, seminar or conference.
- College/university courses taken on campus.
- College/university courses taken remotely.
- Live, multi-location, interactive audio/video instruction originating from within or outside of the organization
- Mentoring, that is, an extended one-on-one confidential relationship focused on meeting the mentee's needs.
- Tutoring or coaching, that is special help from the organization's personnel or outside experts in mastering prescribed skills or material. "Outside expert" could mean a colleague, consultant, or vendor.
- Rotating personnel to encourage learning and cross training.
- Preparing, using and continuously improving written guidelines (sometimes called best practices, procedures, tips, checklists) for frequently used technical and non-technical processes. Written guidelines are initially drafted by experienced personnel and

then frequently updated and refined by other personnel who use the guidelines. While an initial major effort is needed to prepare written guidelines, long-term benefits include E&T, increased productivity, continuous improvement, elimination of valueless activities, and reduced errors and omissions.

Native ability without education
is like a tree without fruit.

— Samuel Johnson

Consider hiring a pharmacist or pharmacy technician to lead a department E&T program. This may be in addition to someone, perhaps from human resources, to administer the E&T program on a part-time or full-time basis.

▢ E&T is often viewed as a program to be cut whenever fiscal, time utilization, or other difficulties arise.

▢ Assume the department/organization is truly committed to E&T. Then pharmacy leadership can help to bridge difficult times by being a knowledgeable advocate for the E&T program within the highest levels of the organization.

▢ The credibility of the organization's principals who advocate E&T will be tested during difficult times. Personnel will judge the organization's commitment to E&T by what the principals do during difficult times, not by what they previously said.

Continuing competence will require continued
learning, unlearning, and relearning.

— Max D. Ray

Include on-going evaluation and support measures in the E&T program

- ■ Continuously assess the quality of the program with emphasis on the extent to which newly learned material is being applied, or at least tried. Accountability will provide a return on the investment in E&T. Absent accountability, the results will be disappointing. Consider using evaluation and support approaches such as the following:

  - Pre-and post-E&T event exams to determine if new knowledge and skills are being acquired as a result of the events, although not necessarily used.

  - End-of-workshop or other E&T event evaluations to obtain participant views on topics such as pre-event information and coordination, meeting room and other physical arrangements, usefulness of presented material, value of handouts, and presenter/facilitator effectiveness.

  - Anecdotes that illustrate the successful application of newly acquired knowledge or skills. Use newsletters, meetings and other means to share the anecdotes. While accounts of interesting incidents may not prove anything, their personal and specific nature raises awareness and encourages fresh thinking.

  - Post-workshop or other E&T event evaluation by supervisors conducted about 2 weeks after the event to determine if personnel are at least trying to apply recently obtained knowledge and skills.

  - Anonymous 360-degree evaluations of supervisors and managers to determine their support of and contributions to the organization's E&T effort.

  - Trends in key indicators such as turnover rate, benchmarking comparisons, absence rates, recruitment costs, patient satisfaction, employee satisfaction, interdepartmental satisfaction, and operating margin profitability.

  - Recognition of individuals who successfully complete E&T events or programs. For example, provide certificates of completion, award continuing education units, send congratulatory letters to the homes of personnel, publish articles in organizational newsletters, and place notes in personnel files.

~~~~~~~~~~~~~~~~~~~~~~~~~~~~~~~

Are you green and growing,

or ripe and rotting.

— Ray Kroc

Read the following related lessons

▫ Lessons 19 through 24 in Part 3, "Teaching and Learning"

▫ Lesson 38, "Our Most Important Asset"

Refer to one or more of the following supplemental sources

▫ Nimmo CM. *Staff Development for Pharmacy Practice.* Bethesda, MD: American Society of Health-System Pharmacists; 2000.

▫ The Health Care Communication Group. *Writing, Speaking, and Communication Skills for Health Care Professionals.* Yale University Press. 2001.

▫ Elliott DP, Burke KW, Lorenzo AG, Hess JA. Drug information course for pharmacy staff development. *Am J Health-Syst Pharm.* 1992;49:2935–2938.

▫ Seo TH, Udeh EC. Videotape programs for pharmacists staff development. *Am J Health-Syst Pharm.* 2003;60:691–693.

▫ Massaro FJ, Harrison MR, Soares A. Use of problem-based learning in staff training and development. *Am J Health-Syst Pharm.* 2006;63:2256–2259.

▫ Marshall JM, Adams JP, Janich JA. Practical, ongoing competency-assessment program for hospital pharmacists and technicians. *Am J Health-Syst Pharm.* 1997;54:1412–1417.

▫ Craig SA, Clark T. Professional development and continuing education programs for pharmacists in large hospitals. *Am J Health-Syst Pharm.* 1988;45: 2503–2506.

▫ Salverson SM, Murante LJ. Clinical training program based on a practice change model. *Am J Health-Syst Pharm.* 2002;59:862–866.

◘ Brouker ME, Mallon TA, Barbour PJ. In-house clinical training program for staff pharmacists. *Am J Health-Syst Pharm.* 1997;54:1794, 1797.

◘ Keith MR, Coffey EL. Clinical training program for distributive pharmacists. *Am J Health-Syst Pharm.* 1997;54:674–677.

The mind is not a vessel to be filled but a fire to be kindled.

— Plutarch

Part 4

|||||||||||||||||||||||||||||||||||||||||||||||||||||||||||||||||||||||||

Improving Personal and Organizational Productivity

Success inevitably comes our way as we acquire, develop, and apply management and leadership knowledge, skills and attitudes, like those suggested and illustrated in this book. With the exhilaration of success, especially the success of doing significant work and making meaningful contributions, comes the realization that we, as individuals and organizations could achieve much more. We are surrounded by an ever-growing galaxy of varied and exciting opportunities and possibilities. We may find ourselves saying, "so much to do, so little time."

While working harder may be the answer to exploring newer opportunities and pursuing new possibilities, working smarter is likely to be smarter. This section offers advice on ways to improve personal and organizational productivity so that we can accomplish more. Suggestions range from more awareness and effective use of our subconscious mind to strengthening project management.

We Don't Make Whitewalls: Work Smarter, Not Harder

||||||||||||||||||||||||||||||||||||||||||||||||||||||||||||||||||||||||||||||||||

We know where most of the creativity,

the innovation,

the stuff that drives productivity lies—

in the minds of those closest to the work.

— Jack Welch

How many times have we received or given the "work smarter, not harder" advice that appears as the subtitle of this lesson? Ten times, one hundred times, or a thousand times? Whatever our answer, I suspect that it will be one or two orders of magnitude greater than the number of times the advice was heeded.

Nonetheless, the advice is both simple and sound. While most of us are willing to work hard and to make whatever effort is needed to get a job done, few would quarrel with the concept of working smarter. After all, working smarter implies benefits such as putting in fewer hours to complete tasks, increasing personal time, incurring less stress, obtaining results that are more likely to meet expectations, and increasing profits.

So why do we repeatedly fail to take our own advice? I see two reasons for this, that is, two obstacles to following what we know to be simple and sound advice. First, we often lack the will or self-discipline to make the up-front investment in time and energy needed to examine the way we do things, either individually or as a group, and to determine if there may be a better way. Time always seems to be a precious commodity. Carving out sufficient time to, in effect, study the way we spend our time is difficult.

Secondly, and more troubling, we recognize consciously or subconsciously that if we truly examine how we do what we do we are very likely to find needed improvements. These improvements will require change and change is difficult.

In the interest of working smarter, not harder, please consider trying one of the following two suggestions. First, at the personal level, set aside some quality time. Think about one work-related process that you frequently do by yourself, or largely by yourself. Examples might be planning, conducting and following up on a meeting of a committee you chair; writing a monthly report; or giving a talk. Search for ways to do it smarter. This may require consultation with selected colleagues. An analysis of how smart we work as individuals, contrasted with how many hours we work, might bear fruit. According to teacher, author and motivational speaker Bill Fitzpatrick[1]:

> Some people actually work as little as half the time they are at work. These people create a window of opportunity for you to succeed. Don't worry about being obligated to work more hours to beat the competition. You probably don't have to. Instead, if you commit to working all the time you are at work, you will probably come out well ahead of your competition.

The second working smarter suggestion involves an ad hoc group effort. Facilitate a work session of predetermined duration within your work place. Select some routine process regularly done by a group of personnel. Examples are assembling a policy and procedure, designing a medication use evaluation, preparing a patient satisfaction survey, or creating a proposal for a new pharmacy service. An interdepartmental process is preferred.

Gather a cross section of individuals who have some role, even if it appears minor, in the process. If, for example, the process is designing a medication use evaluation, don't assemble a group on only pharmacists. Include all players such as technicians, nurses, and physician staff. Establish a non-threatening atmosphere by prohibiting overly critical comments on ideas that are offered. Encourage everyone to participate on an equal basis.

Ask the group to construct a flow chart or some other detailed description of the selected process. Refer to this as the "as is" situation. Then, brainstorm ways to collectively work smarter to create a more effective process. Implement the changes, at least a portion of them, on a trial basis.

Group efforts such as this are successful because each member of the group stands to benefit from the improvements. There are three additional reasons:

- Most people want to contribute to a team effort.
- Non-threatening group efforts are typically very creative and synergistic.
- Individuals closest to a process are in the best position to improve it.

If the preceding ad hoc group effort intrigues you and others, then explore the possibility of conducting a formal review of how routine processes get done. This approach, which is commonly called reengineering,[2] seeks increased efficiency while maintaining or enhancing quality.

Mastering the concept of working smarter, not harder, requires discipline and courage to look inward—within yourself and your organization. Valuable beds of knowledge underlay your organization, but must be sought out, mined and used.[3] Knowledge management authors, Carla O'Dell and C. Jackson Grayson, Jr. observe that "cave dwellers froze to death on beds of coal. Coal was right under them, but they couldn't see it, mine it or use it." In a similar fashion, the typical public or private organization is underlain by valuable beds of knowledge. And like the cave dwellers, if those organizations don't search for, mine and use that knowledge, they may "freeze to death."

Don't tell me how hard you work.
Tell me how much you get done.

— James Ling

Suggestions for Applying Ideas

Read the following story and consider whether unexamined wasteful practices occur within your organization

■ An ambitious and inquisitive worker starts a new production line job at a tire manufacturing plant. After 1 week, he conscientiously asks why each tire is wrapped in brown paper before shipping. His supervisor's answer: "To protect the whitewalls." The new workers response: "We don't make whitewalls, the plant stopped doing that 10 years ago."

■ Are you still wrapping tires in brown paper or its equivalent?

Never mistake motion for action.

— Ernest Hemingway

Avoid thinking that reorganization is the only option for solving organizational problems

■ An organization is a team, or perhaps a group of teams. The three team essentials are a strong and shared commitment to a goal, if not a vision; diversity, that is, an optimum mix of players covering all the necessary bases; and an effective operational structure.

■ Therefore, recognize that reorganizing, or reorganizing again, addresses only the last of the three-team essentials. Before reorganizing, ask if the cause of the problem, and therefore, the solution to, unsatisfactory results might lie instead with lack of goals and/or commitment to them or be traced to misfit players.

I was to learn later in life that
we tend to meet any situation by reorganizing;
a wonderful method it can be
for creating the illusion of progress
while producing confusion, inefficiency
and demoralization.

— Petronius

- Individuals are often the root cause of poor performance, just as they are frequently the source of exemplary performance. In the former case, they should have an opportunity to receive critiques of their behavior and possibly change it and their performance. When the performance or behavior of one or a few individuals is deteriorating or unacceptable, there is a tendency to reorganize the affected unit or even the entire organization. This shotgun approach is sometimes taken in lieu of the rifle approach of personally confronting the problem person or personnel.

Apply some of Og Mandino's success secrets, which help each of us work smarter and wiser[4]

- "Form good habits and become their slaves."
- Respect ourselves and, as a result, "zealously inspect" whatever may enter our bodies, minds, souls and hearts."
- Persist until we succeed never allowing a day to end in failure.
- Appreciate our individual uniqueness and recognize that none of us is "on this earth by chance," each of us should search for our unique purpose.

- Master our emotions recognizing that "unless my mood is right the day will be a failure."

- Aim high always striving to improve recognizing that "to surpass the deeds of others is unimportant; to surpass my own deeds is all."

- Act now, recognizing that dreams, plans, and goals are worthless without action.

～～～～～～～～～～～～～～～～～～～

In truth, the only difference between those who have failed,
and those who have succeeded
lies in the difference of their habits.
Good habits are the key to all success…
I will form good habits and become their slave.

— Og Mandino

Get past the gatekeepers by trying some "work smarter" tactics

"Gatekeepers" are those sometimes overly protective administrative assistants and others who may prevent you from talking by telephone with a key person.[5]

- Call early or late; "bosses" often start work early in the day and are among the last to leave at the end of the day.

- Ask the gatekeeper to help you set up a definite time for a telephone meeting as an alternative to you repeatedly calling on the chance that you will connect.

- Leave an intriguing message, via voicemail with the gatekeeper. I once left this voicemail message. "I have a $1000 opportunity." The person quickly called back. However, the opportunity was a request to have his organization donate $1000 to a professional society.

- Mention a third party known to the person you are trying to contact by telephone. For example, "Mary Jones suggested that I call you to discuss your pharmacy automation needs." However, do this only if the referral is absolutely legitimate.

Adopt the seven habits of highly successful people to help you work smarter[6]

- ◻ Be proactive
- ◻ Begin with the end in mind
- ◻ Put first things first
- ◻ Think win/win
- ◻ Seek first to understand, then to be understood
- ◻ Synergize
- ◻ Sharpen the saw (i.e., renew our physical, spiritual, mental, and social/emotional dimensions).

Avoid continuing or adopting the seven habits of highly ineffective people[7]

- ◻ Poor listening
- ◻ Negative thinking
- ◻ Disorganization
- ◻ Inappropriateness (i.e., failing to recognize that there is a time and place for everything)
- ◻ Decisions by default
- ◻ Randomization (i.e., performing tasks in random order rather than in logical sequence)
- ◻ Procrastination.

Leverage the work already completed or committed to—a little investment on the margin could realize a large return on the margin

- ◻ Your department just implemented a decision support tool to guide physicians prescribing to meet the CMS SCIP quality indicators. Possible small incremental investment: co-author a paper on the project with your group and present findings at the Medical Executive Committee. Possible large incremental return: recognition for the high-level role pharmacists play in the organization and increased resource allocation to fund more projects.

◫ You are well known for putting together coherent, thorough business plans for new clinical services. Many coworkers ask for your help in reviewing their business plans but this is a time consuming endeavor. Possible small incremental investment: prepare a short presentation and handout of how to construct business plans and elements required and share with your coworkers in a workshop or management retreat. Possible large incremental return: reduce requests for reviews of plans, build strong relationships, and increase the functioning of your organization.

◫ You are assembling a presentation to students and residents regarding leadership in the pharmacy profession. Possible small incremental investment: invite staff pharmacists or technicians, to attend on the premise that most people like to learn. Possible large incremental return: improved relations and an increased interest on the part of the staff in leadership activities.

◫ The "i's" have been dotted and the "t's" crossed; copies of your department's annual report are about to be disseminated to the department's coordinators and managers. Possible small incremental investment: hand deliver the reports. While there, thank your coordinators and his/her staff for their work throughout the year. Possible large incremental return: an extra measure of appreciation, on behalf of the coordinators and staff, for being appreciated.

◫ Consider some of your or your organization's recent accomplishments. You understandably want to move on to other projects. However, before doing so, might there be ways in which you can creatively leverage your efforts?

Read the following related lessons

◫ Lesson 3, "Smart Goals"

◫ Lesson 24, "Education and Training: From Ad Hoc to Bottom Line"

◫ Lesson 27, "Delegation: Why Put Off Until Tomorrow What Someone Else Can Do Today?"

◫ Lesson 28, "TEAM: Together Everyone Achieves More"

◫ Lesson 29, "Virtual Teams"

■ Lesson 42, "AH HA! A Process for Effecting Change"

Study one or more of the following sources cited in this lesson

1. Fitzpatrick B. *100 Action Principles of the Shaolin*. Natick, MA: American Success Institute; 1997.

2. Hammer M, Stanton SA. *The Reengineering Revolution: A Handbook*. New York: Harper Collins; 1995.

3. O'Dell C, Grayson CJ, Jr. *If Only We Knew What We Know*. New York: The Free Press; 1998: ix.

4. Mandino O. *The Greatest Salesman in the World*. New York: Bantam Books; 1989.

5. Grugal R. Get past the gatekeepers. *Investors Business Daily*. October 22, 2002.

6. Covey SR. *The 7 Habits of Highly Effective People*. New York: Simon & Schuster; 1989.

7. Green L. The 7 habits of highly ineffective people. *American Way*. August 15, 1995:56–60.

Find the essence of each situation,
like a logger clearing a log jam.
The pro climbs a tall tree and locates the key log,
blows it, and lets the stream do the rest.
An amateur would start at the edge of the jam
and move all the logs,
eventually moving the key log.
Both approaches work, but the "essence" concept saves
time and effort.
Almost all problems have a "key" log if we learn to find it.

— Fred Smith

Lesson 26

The Power of Our Subconscious

||||||||||||||||||||||||||||||||||||||||||||||||||||||||||||||||||||||||||||||||

A man cannot directly choose his circumstances,
but he can choose his thoughts,
and so indirectly, yet surely,
shape his circumstances.

— James Allen

Writing and leadership are similar in that we often "run into a brick wall" in both cases. In the case of writing, the "wall" often appears when we know what we want to say but can't find the words to do it. The leadership "wall" looms when we first truly understand all the constraints and expectations for a project but can't see a way to even come close to satisfying them. Often times, "out of the blue," appear the words or the way.

Psychiatrist and author M. Scott Peck[1] calls the mysterious source and force our unconscious mind. He says, "The conscious mind makes decisions and translates them into actions. The unconscious mind resides below the surface, it is the possessor of extraordinary knowledge that we aren't naturally aware of."

Motivational author Napoleon Hill[2] devoted decades of studying successful people and has this to say about the subconscious mind: "your subconscious mind works continuously, while you are awake and while you sleep." He also suggests that our subconscious mind can actually be directed to work for us:

> The subconscious mind will translate into physical equivalent, by the most direct and practical methods available, any order which is given to it in a state of belief, or faith that that order will be carried out.

As a Man Thinketh, by James Allen,[3] refers to the power of the mind as a "garden, which may be intelligently cultivated or allowed to run wild"; regardless of whether the mind is cultivated or neglected, it will "bring forth." Allen goes on to say that "thought-forces and mind-elements operate in the shaping" of a person's "character, circumstances, and destiny." In other words, we tend to become what we repeatedly say to ourselves we are.[4] So talk to yourself, but be careful what you say; it is very likely to come true.

In his book, *The Power of your Subconscious Mind,*[5] theologian and scientist Joseph Murphy portrays the subconscious mind as being receptive, impressionable, sleepless, non-reasoning, creative, eager, action or execution oriented, intelligent, idea rich, and ageless. Murphy explains: "If you imagine an objective clearly, you will be provided with the necessities, in ways you know not of, through the wonder-working of your subconscious mind."

*Worry consists of creating mental pictures
of what you do not want to happen.
Confidence is creating mental pictures
of what you want to happen.*

— John C. Maxwell

What has this to do with pharmacy managing and leading? The subconscious mind is a powerful tool for working through difficult problems in our professional or personal lives. Rather than physically plug it in and forcefully apply it to the task at hand, we can relax and let it work in the background, creatively, within us. The answers we seek, the options we try—all will come forward.

Suggestions for Applying Ideas

Understand and appreciate the workings of conscious and subconscious minds using these analogies and metaphors

- ▢ The conscious mind is the camera and the subconscious mind is the film.[5] Point your "camera" at the things you want to develop.

- ▢ The conscious mind sees reality while the subconscious mind cannot tell the difference between reality seen by the conscious mind or that which is imagined by the conscious mind.[6] Therefore, consciously imagine and visualize those good things you desire and your subconscious mind will accept and work on them as though they were an evolving reality.

- ▢ The conscious mind selects and plants seeds and the subconscious mind germinates and grows them. Select seeds in accordance with what you want to harvest.[5]

- ▢ If the conscious mind, exercising its free choice selects a worthy direction, the subconscious mind, directed by providence, directs the step.[7]

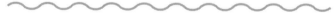

Our life is what our thoughts make it.

— Marcus Aurelius

- ▢ The subconscious mind is an empty file folder, the conscious mind is the filer. Sift and winnow that which appears in your in basket and file only that which you intend to act on.

- ▢ Your conscious mind is the cause; your subconscious mind, the effect. Choose your causes carefully.[5]

▧ The conscious mind is a part-time worker while the subconscious mind is a full-time worker; it never sleeps.[5] Use the limited time available with your conscious mind to direct and fully utilize the continuous, creative efforts of your subconscious mind.

▧ The conscious mind is the ship's captain and the subconscious mind a fast ship and with an excellent crew.[5]

▧ The conscious mind is the front burner, where attention is focused. The subconscious mind is the back burner using a process that "mixes, blends and simmers ingredients into a tasty meal."[8] Feed the back burner of your mind with a "list of problems, facts, and variables, and possible solutions." Let them simmer and expect a pleasing result.

The greatest discovery of my generation is that man can alter his life simply by altering his attitude of mind.

— William James

Use Hill's technique for realizing the potential of your subconscious mind[2,4]

▧ Avoid idle wishing, instead use your conscious mind to specifically define in words, images, and feelings, what you want to accomplish and when. For example, if you are engaged in a writing project, define the message you want to communicate and the responses you want to elicit. If you are designing a new pharmacy clinical service, define the constraints and expectations. Envision the thoughts, words and actions of the eventual uses of your service.

▧ Reduce that well-defined desire to writing which will further clarify your desire and embed it in your mind's eye.

▧ Temporarily set the project aside and have faith that your subconscious mind will go to work on it.

▧ Study, observe, network, ask, imagine, experiment, risk, persist and be positive, not necessarily with your desire in mind, but to serve as stimuli for your subconscious mind.

⬚ Occasionally consciously revisit your project and be prepared to see new ideas which emerge from the work your subconscious mind has been doing and enable you to take steps towards achieving that which you desire.

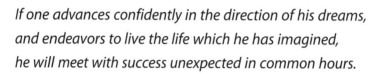

If one advances confidently in the direction of his dreams,
and endeavors to live the life which he has imagined,
he will meet with success unexpected in common hours.

— Henry David Thoreau

Let your subconscious mind work while you sleep

⬚ Try using your subconscious mind during sleep as suggested by inventor Ray Kurzweil, whose creations include the Kurzweil Reading Machine for the blind "which converts ordinary books, magazines, and other printed material to speech."[9]

⬚ Before going to sleep, think about a specific issue or problem, professional or otherwise.

⬚ Don't try to resolve the issue or solve the problem. Instead carefully define it and think of attributes of the resolution or solution.

⬚ Your subconscious mind may be stimulated to work on the problem while you sleep. The dream state is not bound by the restrictions we typically place on our conscious thoughts.

⬚ On awakening, immediately recall the issue or problem and look for new insights or even a resolution of the issue or solution to the problem.

In human affairs
the willed future always prevails
over the logical future.

— Rene Dubos

Read the following related lessons

- Lesson 2, "Roles, Then Goals"
- Lesson 3, "Smart Goals"
- Lesson 25, "We Don't Make Whitewalls: Work Smarter, Not Harder"

If the desire to get something is strong enough in a person,
his whole being, conscious and unconscious,
is always at work,
looking for and devising means to get to the goal.

— Frederick Philip Grove

Study one or more of the following sources cited in this lesson

1. Peck MS. *The Road Less Traveled and Beyond: Spiritual Growth in an Age of Anxiety.* New York: Simon & Schuster; 1997.

2. Hill N. *Think and Grow Rich.* New York: Fawcett Crest Book; 1960.

3. Allen J. *As a Man Thinketh.* White Plains, NY: Peter Pauper Press; 1983.

4. Singleton M. Programming your subconscious mind for success. *Executive Journal.* June 1990: 8–14.

5. Murphy J. *The Power of Your Subconscious Mind.* Englewood Cliffs, NJ: Prentice-Hall; 1963.

6. Tice L. Winners circle network with Lou Tice. An e-newsletter from

the Pacific Institute, (http://www.thepacificinstitute.com); April 25, 2002.

7. Proverbs 16:9, Bible, Good News Version, "You may make your plans but God directs your actions."

8. Carlson R. *Don't Sweat the Small Stuff … and It's All Small Stuff.* New York: Hyperion; 1997.

9. Mink M. Inventor Ray Kurzweil: his passion to create helped give blind people their independence. *Investors Business Daily.* July 10, 2001.

The greatest achievement was at first
and for a time a dream.
The oak sleeps in the acorn;
the bird waits in the egg;
and in the highest vision of the soul a working angel stirs.
Dreams are the seedlings of realities.

— James Allen

Delegation: Why Put Off Until Tomorrow What Someone Else Can Do Today?

Good managers never put off until tomorrow what they can get someone else to do today.

— Anonymous

Delegation, by definition, is legitimately and carefully assigning part of our tasks to someone else, and we pharmacists typically dislike delegation. As part of the deal, we must give up some authority while retaining responsibility for the outcome. Delegation is different from "dumping," that is, getting rid of responsibility when the going gets tough. Delegation is also not giving orders, that is, holding back authority, while giving someone else responsibility.

Collectively, and sometimes even individually, our "can't or won't" delegate reasons are numerous. For example, we can't find the time for the up-front investment needed to show someone how to do what we do. Or no onc could possibly "do it" as well as we do or, maybe they could, but we have no one to delegate to. Another reason is while we know how to do what we do, we lack the organizational and communication skills to explain it to others. Fear of losing knowledge-based job security is a factor for some of us. Others are wary of appearing lazy or incompetent. And, sometimes we hesitate to delegate because we fear advancement. That is, you are concerned that effective delegation may lead to rapid advancement to a more responsible position for which you do not feel prepared.

Frankly, I've heard all the "can't or won't" delegate reasons or, more likely rationalizations, and have used many myself. You may convince yourself but not others, especially peers and those who determine your salary, bonuses, and promotions. Why? Because the reasons to delegate far outweigh the reasons not to. Consider these benefits of delegation[1]:

- ▣ *Frees up experienced people* to take on new responsibilities, projects, and challenges—to do things they are better prepared for or would rather do.

- ▣ Gives other members of the organization *opportunities to learn, grow, and contribute* in new ways to the work of the organization.

- ▣ Helps individuals *learn from others* with, surprisingly, the learning sometimes flowing from the delegatees to delegators.

- ▣ *Reduces task costs*, that is, it tends to push the cost of each task to the lowest level possible consistent with the required results.

- ▣ *Builds resiliency* into an organization. By spreading understanding of tools and techniques to other members of the organization, more people know how to do more things. This is analogous to the concept of "strengthening the bench" on an athletic team.

If you are still in the "can't or won't" category then recognize that the usual consequence of not delegating within an organization is that you are likely to be relegated to the slow track. Failure to delegate will probably label you as "not being a people person" and "not being a team player" and stymie both managerial and technical advancement. In contrast, through delegation you help your colleagues and organizations realize some of the previously listed benefits. You demonstrate many important management and leadership perspectives and skills, not the least of which is teamwork.

I not only use all the brains I have,
but all I can borrow.

— Woodrow Wilson

Suggestions for Applying Ideas

Follow these tips for successful delegation[1, 2]

- Make sure you understand your responsibility and have the authority to carry it out. Typically some project or process has been delegated to you and you, in turn, are delegating a portion of it to someone else.

- Explain the context for the delegated task. For example, describe the overall process or project and indicate how the delegated task fits in terms of inputs and outputs.

- Use written procedures which may also be called checklists, tips, guidelines or best practices. Ask the delegatee to suggest improvements to the written procedures.

- Provide, as may be appropriate, the resources available and schedule for the task. Rather than using a single completion date, the schedule could be presented as a series of milestone dates with portions of the task being completed by each milestone.

- Prescribe and illustrate expected outcomes and deliverables. Use factors such as accuracy, format, size, and customer satisfaction.

- Provide or arrange for the necessary tools and resources.

- Do not over-prescribe "how." Avoid giving orders and micro-managing.

- Protect the delegatee from outside intrusions, well intentioned or otherwise.

- Recognize these three possible outcomes of delegation, arranged from favorable to unfavorable, and respond accordingly:

  - The work is delivered as needed.

- The work will not be completed as needed but the delegator is so advised by the delegatee well before the deadline.

- The work is not going to be completed as expected, and the delegator learns about the deficiency at or after the time the work was to be completed.

☐ When the outcome meets or exceeds expectations, say "thank you" in a way that clearly communicates what you appreciate and why. As noted by fiction writer and humorist, Mark Twain, "I can live for two months on a good compliment."

☐ If the outcome is unsatisfactory, take action. Critique the work, not the person; avoid negative "you" messages. Hold the delegatee accountable for meeting his or her responsibility. Look for ways that the delegatee can partly or completely correct the unsatisfactory outcome.

A real leader does as much dog work for his people as he can: he can do it, or see a way to do without it, ten times as fast. And he delegates as many important matters as he can because that creates a climate in which people grow.

— Robert Townsend

Test yourself for delegation effectiveness by answering the following questions "yes" or "no"

☐ Are you working longer hours than almost everyone else?

☐ Do you regularly take work home?

☐ Are you frequently rushing to meet deadlines?

☐ Are top priority action items needed to fill your desired roles and achieve your established goals on the "back burner" or, worse yet, not even started?

☐ Are you the only person capable of managing the next big assignment or project?

□ Is your staff listless and stagnant and/or do you experience high turnover?

If most or all of your answers are "yes" you are fooling and shortchanging yourself, others and your organization.[2]

Take your delegation effectiveness up to a new level by following these suggestions

□ Think of a task that "only you can do." Plan to delegate it, or part of it, to someone else.

□ Plan to delegate a task to someone you have never delegated to.

□ Try one more time to delegate a task to someone who failed in the past. Maybe you were part of the problem.

□ Urge one of your non-delegating supervisees to try delegation.

□ Identify someone from whom you will no longer accept substandard performance. Hold them accountable to meet his or her responsibility the next time they come up short.

Identity requires responsibility
because without responsibility there is no self respect.
You do not know whether you could handle anything,
deliver any result or take care of anyone else.

— Charles Handy

□ Think of someone who always comes through when tasks are delegated—who does it so well, that you hardly notice. Say "thank you," recalling the earlier advice to be very specific.

Read the following related lessons

□ Lesson 22, "More Coaching, Less Osmosis"

■ Lesson 25, "We Don't Make Whitewalls: Work Smarter, Not Harder"

■ Lesson 38, "Our Most Important Asset"

Study one or more of the following sources cited in this lesson

1. Walesh SG. Management of relationships. In *Engineering Your Future: The Non-Technical Side of Professional Practice in Engineering and Other Technical Fields.* 2nd ed. Chapter 4. Reston, VA: ASCE Press; 2000.

2. Culp G, Smith A. Six steps to effective delegation. *Journal of Management in Engineering–ASCE;* January/February 1997: 30–31.

Irrevocable commitments that offer no loopholes, no bailout provisions, and no parachute clauses will extract incredible productivity and performance.

— Robert A. Schuller

TEAM: Together Everyone Achieves More

One hand cannot applaud alone.

— Arabian proverb

The implementation of a new pharmacy computer system involves extensive work to prepare the system for use followed by an organized team effort at "go-live." The launch involves training staff on use of the new system and then transitioning all existing patient information from the old system to the new system. Ideally the transfer of data is an electronic process, but in many cases it requires keyboard re-entry of the patient's medication profile. Our recent go-live required the latter, which was extremely labor intense. We were fortunate that the go-live was well-planned and orchestrated as it involved nearly 50% of our pharmacist staff and took the better part of a weekend. The effort of managers, coordinators, pharmacists, residents and students was a tremendous team effort that went extremely well.

Involvement of staff in community service activities can be a very rewarding addition to the day to day routine of a pharmacy staff. Our health system is a major sponsor of the American Heart Walk in our city. Members of our department are extremely proud of the annual contribution of the "Pharmacy Family Heart Walk Team." For each of the past three years, the pharmacy team has raised the most money of any department in the health system and ranked within the top ten teams in city. This is a great accomplishment when the number of staff in the department compared to other much larger departments is considered.

What teamwork lesson can we learn from successful group experiences like the two cited here? I am convinced that the three key elements of successful teamwork are:

- ☒ A strong and shared commitment to an ambitious **vision;** the bolder the better. The litmus test: The vision should initially appear highly desirable but unachievable.

- ☒ **Diversity;** an optimum mix of players. All the necessary bases must be covered. Factors to consider in forming a team are to seek individuals who, besides sharing the vision, collectively bring the necessary knowledge, skills, connections, and time availability.

- ☒ An effective operational **structure.** Trust and open, on-going, intra-team communication are essential.

All three elements are needed, none is sufficient. An exciting vision without diverse players is a dream. A talented team toiling in a vision void is poor stewardship. Engineer and educator Arthur E. Morgan said "Lack of something to feel important about is almost the greatest tragedy a man may have."[1] A superb organizational structure without talented players degenerates into bureaucracy.

Architect and city planner Daniel Burnham suggested the power of vision-driven teamwork when he said, "Make no little plans, they have no magic to stir men's blood. Make big plans, aim high in hope and work and let your watchword be order and your beacon beauty."

Great discoveries and improvements invariably
involve the co-operation of many minds.
I may be given credit for having blazed the trail
but when I look at the subsequent developments
I feel the credit is due to others rather than to myself.

— Alexander Graham Bell

Suggestions for Applying Ideas

Perform reality checks

- ◘ Have you, in your work, community, athletic, family or other endeavors, recently had an uplifting team experience?

- ◘ If not, seek out team opportunities so you don't miss out on one of life's most rewarding experiences.

- ◘ Can you, as a director or manager in your organization, point to outstanding team efforts within your organization?

- ◘ If not, your organization is probably falling far short of its potential. **Suggestion:** Articulate an ambitious vision, assemble a diverse team, ask them to achieve the vision, provide support, and get out of the way.

Appreciate that teams, especially those with ambitious expectations and highly motivated players, often need to progressively work through the four stages of team development[2-4]

1. *Forming*: Politeness, inquiry, waiting to see what will happen, no or very little productivity.

2. *Storming*: Disagreement, confusion, conflict, factions, some productivity.

   The storming stage is not inevitable. It can be reduced in intensity or avoided partly by starting slow, that is, providing opportunities for individuals to become acquainted, providing history and other context for the team's task or charge, developing meeting and communication norms, agreeing on basic terminology, encouraging individuals to share concerns, and defining possible roles of team members.

3. *Norming*: Conflict resolution, goal setting, decision-making, establishment of protocols, ownership, accountability, moderate productivity.

4. *Performing*: Teamwork, adjustments, deliverables, full ownership and accountability, can and will attitude, high productivity, satisfaction, celebration.

*We need leaders who can guide a pharmacy staff
to assume new roles and higher professional responsibilities.*

— Joe E. Smith

Recognize and temper potential "red flags" in team members' personalities[5]

◻ Cynical attitude

◻ Aloofness

◻ Strong need to win

◻ Preference for clearly defined short-term goals and discomfort with ambiguity

◻ Impatience with indecisiveness

◻ Irritability and defensiveness in response to criticism

◻ Meticulousness and intolerance of others' mistakes

◻ Excessive immersion in details

Read the following related lessons

◻ Lesson 29, "Virtual Teams"

◻ Lessons 32 through 34 in "Part 5: Meetings"

Study one or more of the following sources cited in this lesson

1. Leuba CJ. *A Road to Creativity–Arthur Morgan–Engineer, Educator, Administrator.* North Quincy, MA: Christopher Publishing House; 1971.

2. Brown TL. Teams can work great. *Industry Week;* February 1992: 18.

3. Krumberger JM. Group facilitation: building that winning team. *Nursing Dynamics.* 1992: 1(3):9

4. Martin P, Tate K. Climbing to performance. *PM Network;* June 1999: 14.

5. Thompson JW. Engineers don't always make the best team players. *Electronic Engineering Times;* September 30, 1996: 124.

Refer to the following supplemental sources

▪ Hardingham A, Ellis C. *The Ultimate Team Building Toolkit: 32 Exercises for Trainers.* New York: American Management Institute; 2002.

This book enables teams, and those who coach teams, to engage in "just-in-time" learning. It provides structured exercises both for developing a team's general capability to work together and also for developing their repertoire of specific team working tools and techniques.

▪ Shonk JH. *Team-Based Organizations: Developing a Successful Team Environment.* Chicago, IL: Irwin Professional Publishing; 1997.

Builds on the premise that teams offer "an effective way to coordinate across organizational boundaries in solving problems and gaining employee commitment." Intended for managers and leaders, this book explains how to plan for and implement transitioning an organization from a traditional hierarchical and functional structure to more team-based organization.

Visit one or more of these websites

▪ "About Teambuilding, Inc." (http://www.teambuildinginc.com) is offered by a participatory management consulting firm led by civil engineer Peter Grazier. Many free, team-related articles are offered. Another useful feature is a discussion section where visitors can post questions for response by Grazier and others.

▪ "Team Management Systems" (http://www.tms.com.au), is maintained by Australian consultants, whose firm focuses on "why some individuals, teams and organizations perform, work effectively and achieve their objectives, while others fail." Useful free features include many case studies and articles.

*The society which
scorns excellence in plumbing as a humble activity and
tolerates shoddiness in philosophy because it is an exalted activity
will have neither good plumbing nor good philosophy:
neither its pipes nor its theories will hold water.*

— John W. Gardner

Virtual Teams

||||||||||||||||||||||||||||||||||||||||||||||||||||||||||||||||||||||||||||||||||||||||||||||||||

*The diplomatic art of managing
ad hoc partnerships and alliances
will become a key executive skill.*

— *Economist*[1]

With pharmacy experts living across the globe, virtual teams provide a mechanism for these pharmacists to work together to accomplish tasks for the profession. Virtual teams enable these pharmacists to assemble the expertise needed to complete big projects, write guidelines or to take on challenging causes. A virtual team is like a traditional team in that it has the three essentials of common vision or purpose, the necessary diversity of expertise, and an effective structure for communicating and effective working structure. However, in a virtual team, the members typically are a carefully selected, eclectic mix of leaders from various organizations who are usually linked electronically. The explosion of low cost electronic communication devices—email, websites, wireless telephones, PDAs, pagers, and facsimile machines—has facilitated the virtual team phenomenon. An article in the *Economist*[1] draws this conclusion about the business impact of the Internet and other newer technologies:

The boundaries of companies will also change. Companies will find it easier to outsource and to use communications to develop deeper relations with suppliers, distributors and many others who might once have been vertically integrated into the firm.

The legal and organizational structures of the members of a virtual team or organization are secondary. Of prime concern is the extent to which members of the virtual group are able to function in service of the cause. Trust is essential; it is the glue that binds the virtual team or organization.[2]

Virtual teams are increasingly formed to meet the specific and demanding needs of the changing climate of healthcare. Participants recognize that while any one existing organization may not be able to marshal all the necessary talents, a specialty tailored virtual team can do so.

Once the purpose is accomplished, the team is likely to disband never to be re-assembled in exactly the same manner. Some team members may have worked together on virtual teams in the past and others may work together in the future—but only if driven by a cause and by recent compatible, individual performance. Unlike actual teams, virtual teams do not have to "carry" any one because they "need the work" or are on the payroll. There need be no force fits, only perfect fits.

Suggestions for Applying Ideas

Build an effective, functioning virtual team by incorporating these suggestions[3]

▢ "Work only with people you know and trust." Assessing the trustworthiness of a potential team member is difficult but through active participation in national organizations, many good team members will be identified through reputation and previous experience.

▢ Clearly define up front, in writing, and for each team member: the scope of the project, purpose, schedule, deliverables and budget. That is, prepare a project plan and obtain buy-in from all members of the virtual team.

- Establish a communication protocol. For example, select the primary mode of communication recognizing that there are many options including telephone, fax, email, pagers, and websites. With email and website communication, costs are independent of distance, unlike telephone and fax communication. The selection of members for a virtual team and the ease and cost of communication among them should not be hindered by distances among them. Email and website communication supports this principle.

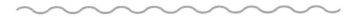

The way a team plays as a whole determines its success.
You may have the greatest bunch of individual stars in the world,
but if they don't play together, the club won't be worth a dime.

— Babe Ruth

Bring a new virtual team together for a face-to-face meeting near the beginning of their work

- Do so even if a team could, from a technical perspective, conduct all of its work via electronic communication.

- As sophisticated and cost effective as electronic communication may be, experience strongly suggests that early minimal, but carefully planned and orchestrated, face-to-face interaction will enhance communication and help to build trust.

- Provide ample opportunity during such face-to-face meetings for casual side conversations.

Be an active, effective participant in conference calls[4]

- If organizing a conference call, express the time in all applicable time zones (e.g., Eastern, Central, Mountain, Pacific). It is very easy for busy professionals to confuse times when participants are in multiple time zones.

- Eliminate distractions. Post a sign on your door instructing people not to interrupt. Do not play music in the background. Do not chew, eat or smoke or do anything that creates noise to distract the participants.

▣ Do not attempt to multitask. All the busy professionals on the call have taken valuable time to work as a group on the project. Working on other issues distracts you from the call and disrupts the group's productivity.

▣ Do not put the call on hold as some telephone systems have music that comes on automatically when you put a call on hold.

▣ Use the mute on your phone whenever you are not talking to reduce distractions.

▣ If you are the moderator and a participant is being noisy you cannot ignore the noise if it interferes with how well the rest of the participants can hear. You should respectfully ask for that participant to call in from another location or ask them to disconnect and state that you will call them back immediately after the call to summarize the results and to get input.

Read the following related lessons

▣ Lesson 15, "Balance High Tech and High Touch"

▣ Lesson 28, "TEAM: Together Everyone Achieves More"

▣ Lessons 32 through 34 in Part 5, "Meetings"

Study one or more of the following sources cited in the lesson

1. When companies connect. *Economist.* June 26, 1999:19–20.

2. King RT. The company we don't keep. *The Wall Street Journal.* November 18, 1996.

3. Ashton A, Ashton R. Long distance relationships. *Home Office Computing.* July 1999:52–55.

4. Lemery LD. Conducting conference calls. *Clinical Leadership & Management Review.* January/February 2002:17–21.

Refer to the following supplemental source

▣ Peters T. Tomorrow's strange enterprises. In *The pursuit of WOW!* New York: Vintage Books; 1994.

Visit one or more of these websites

▣ "Virtual Projects" (http://www.vrtprj.com) is maintained by Rainer Volz, an IT and project management consultant. Features include links to mostly European project management and virtual organization websites and short reviews of project management and virtual team books.

▣ "Livelink Virtualteams" (http://www.virtualteams.com) is maintained by NetAge. Provides many free virtual team articles.

To own resources is a mistake.

Instead, you need instant access to the best resources

from wherever, whenever,

to get the job done…

Now impermanence and improvisation are markers

for success.

— Tom Peters

Fruits of Effective Project Management

||||||||||||||||||||||||||||||||||||||||||||||||||||||||||||||||||||||||||||||||||||||||

Project Management:
The application of knowledge, skills, tools and techniques
to project activities in order to
meet or exceed stakeholder needs and expectations
from a project.

— Project Management Institute

If project management is the tree, then its fruit is the delivery of required products and services, on time and within budget to the satisfaction of the project management team, organization and those we serve. Carefully cultivated and cared for, the project management tree will flourish, bear much fruit, and provide a continuing harvest for an organization and its members. In contrast, if not cared for, the fruits will be diminished in quality and reduced in number.

Project management is a set of processes by which organizations marshal resources to design, develop, implement, and maintain required products and services. The manner in which an organization manages its projects is crucial to satisfying stakeholders. Whether they are large, small, sophisticated, or basic, all projects require careful project management.

The word "project" is used broadly in this lesson. Projects are distinguished from processes in that processes are ongoing and repeated but projects tend to be unique. The Project Management Institute[1] defines a project as:

> A temporary endeavor undertaken to create a unique product or service. Temporary means that every project has a definite beginning and a definite end. Unique means that the product or service is different in some distinguishing way from all similar products or services.

Essentially everyone in an organization, business or otherwise, is at least indirectly involved in projects. Each person can contribute to the successful completion of projects and derive satisfaction from the team's and organization's achievement.

Successful project management propagates throughout an organization, in many and varied positive ways, thus significantly contributing to an organization's success. Conversely, mediocre or failed project management has widespread, negative and sometimes devastating impacts upon an organization. Accordingly, project management should be a major, if not the principal, focus of an organization's energies. Like the trunk of a tree, it is the organization's supporting structure.

There are many fruits of effective project management[2]:

1. ***Happy, satisfied employees and patients.*** Effective project management means quality, that is, meeting requirements. Project management is the activity closest to an organization's employees and patients; they immediately and continuously receive the results, positive or negative, of the way projects are managed.

2. ***Profitability.*** Clearly a business needs profit to survive, let alone thrive, and projects are the profit (or loss) generators.

3. A fantastic on-the-job arena for ***teaching and learning.*** There is no "make believe" here. Individual or organizational capabilities can be markedly enhanced during the conduct of projects. Experience — good and bad — of senior personnel can be readily shared with junior personnel within the project management process.

4. The setting in which existing clinical, technical and business **methods can be improved and new approaches developed.** The idea that "necessity is the mother of invention" is clearly demonstrated in effective project execution.

5. A forum in which individuals and the organization can identify **future needs** of their stakeholders. By following through and meeting those needs, an organization's ability to serve is enhanced.

6. **New projects** with existing stakeholders which enable the team to further develop its capabilities and reputation.

7. The source of ideas, experience, and references from satisfied customers which earn the opportunity to gain more resources and **provide services to an even larger circle of stakeholders.**

8. **Personal satisfaction** through team achievement.

As logical as all the preceding seems to me, and possibly to you, I marvel at the management or, more specifically, the lack of it, of projects. Proven principles and sound steps are routinely ignored. Are you and your organization harvesting your share of the fruits of effective project management?

Suggestions for Applying Ideas

Focus constructively on the three demands of project management

Most projects encounter these three potentially conflicting demands. Satisfying two of the three requirements is easy, but reconciling all three is difficult.

◻ Providing deliverables that satisfy customer and other stakeholder requirements.

◻ Meeting the schedule.

◻ Staying within the budget.

~~~~~~~~~~~~~~~~~~~~~~~~

Project managers fall into three basic categories:

those who watch things happen,

those who make things happen,

and those who wonder what happened.

— Sunny and Kim Baker

Arrange for one member of your team, department, or organization to join the Project Management Institute (PMI) on a 1-year trial basis

- ◻ Review PMI's monthly magazine, *PM Network*; its monthly journal, *Project Management Journal* and the organization's newsletter and selected other publications.

- ◻ Glean and share potentially useful concepts, information, and methodologies in the interest of improving project management. Possibly rotate the reviewing and sharing responsibility among personnel on a monthly basis.

- ◻ The overall thrust is to plug into, on at least an experimental basis, the premier project management professional organization.

Recognize the difference between "project" and "process"

While "project" is used broadly in the lesson, and includes but goes beyond contracted services, not everything we do in our organization is part of a project.[3]

- ◻ "There are only two ways work gets done: through … processes or through projects."

- ◻ "Everything new or improved that happens requires a project. All ongoing operations require … processes."

- ◻ The essentials of projects and processes are listed in Table 30–1

- ◻ When a process is significantly improved or redesigned, that effort becomes a project.

- ◻ Distinguish between projects and processes and manage accordingly.

TABLE 30–1. PROJECT AND PROCESS	
PROJECT	**PROCESS**
Temporary—has a beginning and an end	Ongoing—the same process is repeated over and over again
Produces a unique output or deliverable	Produces the same output each time the process is run
Has no predefined work assignments	Has predefined work assignments

Read the following related lessons

☐ Lesson 28, "TEAM: Together Everyone Achieves More"

☐ Lesson 29, "Virtual Teams"

☐ Lesson 31, "Every Project Is Done Twice"

Study one or more of the following sources cited in this lesson

1. Project Management Institute. *A Guide to the Project Management Body of Knowledge.* 3rd ed. Newtown Square, PA: PMI; 2004.

2. Walesh SG. It's project management, stupid! *Journal of Management in Engineering—ASCE.* January/February 1996:14–17.

3. Martin PK, Tate K. Not everything is a project. *PM Network.* May 2001:25.

Refer to one or more of the following supplemental sources

☐ Baker S, Baker K. *The Complete Idiot's Guide to Project Management.* New York: Alpha Books; 1998.

☐ *Managing Projects Large and Small: The Fundamental Skills for Delivering on Budget and on Time.* Boston: Harvard Business School Press; 2004.

Subscribe to this e-newsletter

◫ "Point Lookout," a free weekly e-newsletter from Chaco Canyon Consulting. Featured are essays and white papers on teamwork, conflict and project management. Many previously published essays and white papers are available at no cost. To subscribe, go to http://www.chacocanyon.com/.

Visit one or more of these websites

◫ "Michael Greer's Project Management Resources" (http://www.michaelgreer.com/) is maintained by consultant Greer whose business offers project management education and training, consulting and products. Offered free are a project management bibliography and many articles including "10 Guaranteed Ways to Screw Up Any Project" and "Project 'Post-mortem' Review Questions."

◫ "The Project Management Institute" (http://www.pmi.org/) is the official website of the 200,000 member PMI. Included are membership information, conference and seminar announcements, calls for papers, and a bookstore.

The road to success
is not doing one thing 100 percent better
but doing 100 things one percent better.

— H. Jackson Brown, Jr.

Every Project Is Done Twice
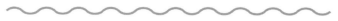

The beginning is the most important part of the work.

— Plato

Organizations that are not satisfied with their project managers' performance take a variety of actions: threaten, offer rewards, reduce the number of project managers, hire or appoint new project managers, provide education and training for and/or certification for project managers, prepare project management handbooks, purchase project management software, and convene gatherings of project managers at which ideas and information are exchanged.

These and other tactics, if carefully selected and optimally combined, can be useful. However, in my view, the most fundamental and powerful "secret" of effective project management is the title of this lesson. Unless project managers are convinced that every project is done twice, and twice in a positive sense, all the threats, treats, training and tools will be of little use.

There is a smart way to do a project twice, and there is a not-so-smart way.[1] The not-so-smart way is wasteful: the first time, the project (or major portions of it) is done wrong because of poor or no planning. Haphazard, high profile, initial activity is viewed as progress. Eventually much of the work has to be redone, that is, done a second time. Negative outcomes typically include waste, frustration, loss of clients or constituents, and, for businesses, low or no profitability.

The smart way to do a project twice is to first mentally create the entire project and then, and only then, *actually* create, that is, execute the project. In other words, plan the work and then work the plan. Think through, then do. This approach requires a high degree of self and organizational discipline. However, it yields a greatly enhanced probability that the second and ultimate creation will be achieved on time and within budget and will meet client and other project requirements.

Careful ingredient selection doesn't assure an excellent dinner and careful preparation of the itinerary doesn't guarantee a memorable trip. However, careful selection of ingredients and careful preparation of the itinerary greatly increase the probability, respectively, of an excellent dinner and a memorable trip. Similarly, careful preparation of a work plan, while it will not guarantee a successful project, will greatly increase the probability of one.

The book *Zen and the Art of Motorcycle Maintenance*,[2] by quality thinker Robert Pirsig, ostensibly describes a process to use for a motorcycle repair project. But his advice is applicable to the many projects underway in our healthcare organizations. Before beginning the project, each of us is urged to do the following:

> List everything you're going to do on little slips of paper, which you then organize into proper sequence. You discover that you organize and then reorganize the sequence again and again as more and more ideas come to you. The time spent that way usually more than pays for itself in time saved on the machine and prevents you from doing fidgety things that create problems later on.

On considering the theme of this lesson, you may be inclined to dismiss it as simple or obvious. Perhaps it is. However, if asked, could you immediately show the written project plan for all of the contract or other projects on which you are the manager or a team member? If project plans exist, have all team members bought into them and are the plans current?

If your answer is "yes" to these questions, you are a rare individual or in a rare organization. And you and your organization are probably harvesting more than your share of project management fruits. If your answer is "no" if you are dissatisfied with your project management yield, maybe a fundamentally new approach is needed. Otherwise, if you do what you did, you'll get what you got.

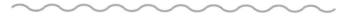

I'll give you a six-word formula for success:
think things through—then follow through.

— Eddie Rickenbacker

Suggestions for Applying Ideas

Include some or all of the following in your project plan

- **Scope of services.** Possibly include or reference a readily available copy of the scope and purpose of the project. Address identification and resolution of scope creep.

- **Team directory.** List key project staff within your organization and possibly other stakeholders within your organization and provide contact information.

- **Communication.** Who are the lead contacts and how and when will they communicate?

- **Work task breakdown.** Identify tasks, related hours and other resources, and responsible individuals.

- **Deliverables and schedule.** Explain what is to be delivered (e.g., report, plan set, cost estimate, meetings) and when.

- **Budget.** Provide a budget (labor and expenses) for each task/individual/department.

- **Written guidelines, checklists, tips, and best practices.** Refer to these documents to avoid reinventing the wheel.

- **Documentation and filing.** Prescribe how meetings, analyses, design and other project tasks will be documented and filed for use during and possibly after the project.

- ◻ **Billing procedure.** Describe procedure and format for and frequency of invoices. Consider including a short status report with each invoice.

- ◻ **Monitoring.** Explain how deliverables, budget and schedule will be monitored and, if needed, modified.

P⁶: Prior proper planning prevents poor performance.

— Anonymous

Try this "low tech" risk assessment method as part of your next project plan[3]

- ◻ Assemble the team that will conduct the project.

- ◻ Give each one sticky notes.

- ◻ Invite team members to brainstorm risks associated with the project, write them on the sticky notes and place them anywhere on newsprint pad, white board, or other readily visible area.

- ◻ Possible potential problems are "physicians don't show up to meetings," "nurses are already learning two other new information systems," and "clinical pharmacists are difficult to recruit."

- ◻ Eliminate duplicates and clarify the meaning of risks as needed.

- ◻ Draw X and Y axes on the newsprint pad, white board or other readily seen area. Write low, medium, and high probability on the Y axis. Write low, medium, and high impact on the X axis.

- ◻ Using group consensus, place the sticky notes on the axes based on their probability and impact.

- ◻ Focus on the high probability—high impact quadrant and brainstorm mitigation measures.

- ◻ Include selected measures in the project plan.

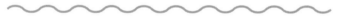

If your project doesn't work,
look for the part
that you didn't think was important.

— Arthur Bloch

Watch for symptoms of the "project plan avoidance syndrome" in yourself and others on the team[4]

- ▫ Solving problems as they arise is more satisfying.
- ▫ Neither time nor environment is available for the focused thinking.
- ▫ Necessary labor is not in the budget.
- ▫ Written project plans provide a means to monitor and measure project manager performance and we fear that evaluation.

Why do we never have enough time to do it right
but always enough time to do it over?

— Anonymous

Read the following related lessons

- ▫ Lesson 28, "TEAM: Together Everyone Achieves More"
- ▫ Lesson 29, "Virtual Teams"
- ▫ Lesson 30, "Fruits of Effective Project Management"

Study one or more of the following sources cited in this lesson

1. Covey SR. *The 7 Habits of Highly Effective People.* New York: Simon & Schuster; 1990.
2. Pirsig RM. *Zen and the Art of Motorcycle Maintenance.* New York: Bantam Books; 1974: 284.

3. Martin PK, Tate K. A project management genie appears. *PM Network.* August 2001:18.

4. Cori KA. Project work plan development. Paper presented at the Project Management Institute and Symposium, October, Atlanta, GA; 1989.

Read the following supplemental sources

■ Rad PF. From the editor. *Project Management Journal.* June 2001: 3. Defines risk management as "the systematic process of identifying, analyzing and responding to a project's unplanned events" and goes on to describe three categories of risks.

■ Managing Projects Large and Small: The Fundamental Skills for Delivering on Budget and on Time. Harvard Business School Publishing Corporation. Harvard Business School Press, Boston Massachusetts; 2004.

The secret of getting ahead is getting started.
The secret of getting started is
breaking your complex overwhelming tasks into
small manageable tasks,
and then starting on the first one.

— Mark Twain

Part 5

‖‖

Meetings

Meetings warrant special attention as a separate section in this book for two reasons. First, as we increase our management and leadership efforts, the number and variety of meetings we orchestrate or are invited to will increase. Increased involvement in meetings can be, on the balance, a positive or negative. That is, synergism happens, ideas flow, decisions occur, commitments are made or our valuable time is wasted, or at least poorly used. What we do before, during, and after meetings determines whether our increased involvement in meetings will be positive or negative, both for ourselves and others.

Second, and this may seem harsh but I believe it to be true, the majority of meetings within pharmacy circles can be better planned, effectively conducted and suffer from poor follow-up. Any one of us can, within our circle of influence, greatly improve meeting effectiveness and create many more positive meeting experiences for all involved.

This section presents simple techniques for enabling a group of diverse individuals with a common purpose to function as a group, to share, debate, create, decide, and act. The suggestions are applicable to traditional, face-to-face meetings; conference calls; and multi-location, audio-video gatherings.

The "Unhidden" Agenda

|||||||||||||||||||||||||||||||||||||||||||||||||||||||||||||||||||||||||||||||||||||

Meetings have become the practical alternative to work.

— Robert Kriegel and David Brandt

The success of most business and other meetings is usually determined before they start. Why? Because pre-meeting planning, especially establishing the content and tone of the agenda, has a major impact on the degree of participation and the quality of the resulting decisions.

Part of the planning should be a conscious decision of whether or not a meeting is needed. Perhaps some other form of communication, such as email exchange, will suffice. When it doubt, don't meet.

Time spent prior to the meeting by the explicitly or implicitly designated leader, preferably assisted by some other likely meeting participants, is the key. Consider the ideas listed below as you prepare the agenda for your next meeting.[1] These suggestions apply to traditional face-to-face meetings as well as conference calls and meetings that combine conference calls for audio with website access for sharing of images.

- ◻ List all the invitees in the "To" portion of the memorandum or email. Knowing who else will attend a meeting can be useful. For example, this information provides an opportunity to informally discuss other matters with one or more individuals immediately before or after the meeting.

▢ Show meeting starting time and ending time on the agenda. This courtesy enables meeting attendees to plan their day, especially the time after this meeting, because they will know when the meeting is to end. A stated and firm ending time also encourages focus and brevity by participants. As noted by psychologists and authors Robert Kriegel and David Brandt,[2] "meetings are a lot like the hot air they produce: they'll expand or contract to fill the space available."

▢ Include the entry "Additional Agenda Items" near the beginning of the agenda. This provides the leader with the opportunity to add topics of discussion and also facilitates input from attendees, some of whom may not have been involved in preparing the original agenda.

▢ Explicitly identify individuals having reporting or other responsibilities. This helps to ensure that they will be prepared to report on their efforts or lead a discussion on the indicated topic.

▢ Attach background, support, and other materials, but don't overdo it. This extra effort by the person managing the meeting arrangements provides participants with the opportunity to be prepared so that the meeting time can be used most effectively.

▢ Establish an action-oriented theme by using words and expressions such as "decide," "select," "follow-up," and "select course of action." In some organizations, such as academic institutions, a meeting might be considered successful if interesting topics are discussed with no decisions made. If the meeting leader wants to avoid this, the agenda should be structured to encourage and expect action.

▢ Suggest, for each agenda item, what participants are expected or encouraged to do. For example, indicate if the group is to develop, discuss, and select alternative solutions to a problem or respond to a recommended course of action developed prior to the meeting by a member of the committee or by others. The person managing arrangements for the meeting diplomatically focuses the energies of the participants. However, recognize that the group may elect to broaden its response to an agenda, but is unlikely to do this if trust is established between the leader and the participants.

◻ Consider adding, depending on the nature of the meeting, an item titled "Good News" under which positive happenings are briefly shared.

Any committee is only as good as the most knowledgeable, determined and vigorous person on it.
There must be somebody who provides the flame.

— Lady Bird Johnson

A proactive invitee can help to effect some of the preceding suggestions. For example if you are invited to a meeting and a written agenda is not provided, ask if an agenda will follow. This may prompt preparation of an agenda and lead to a better meeting. If there will not to be an agenda, insist on knowing what is to be discussed so that you can prepare, decline the invitation, or arrange to have some other, more appropriate person attend in your place.

Assume there is an important point you, as an invited participant, want to make at a meeting, but there is no directly related agenda item. Either you did not have an opportunity to get your concern on the agenda prior to the meeting or the chair was not receptive to adding items at the meeting. Carefully prepare your idea or information. Look for opportunities at the meeting to make your point, perhaps in answer to a question posed to you or to someone else.

Suggestions for Applying Ideas

Evaluate this statement against your experience. There are only two legitimate types of meetings.[1]

◻ **Working meetings.** Agenda items might be problem definitions, presentation and discussion of status reports, brainstorming, conceptualizing options, comparing alternatives, and implementing solutions.

◻ **Briefings on critical non-routine topics**. Examples are personnel matters, reorganization, or serious departmental or patient care issues.

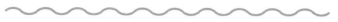

Meetings are indispensable when you don't want to do anything.

— John Kenneth Galbraith

Decide if a meeting is really needed; that is, consider the following reasons *not* to call a meeting[1]

◻ You've made up your mind what to do anyway. Convening others and feigning seeking their counsel wastes everyone's time and risks your credibility.

◻ You know what should be done, but don't want to take responsibility. Therefore, you call a meeting, indicate what should be done, obtain formal approval or informal acquiescence, and then can "spread the blame" if needed.

◻ You don't know what should be done and want somebody else to make the decision. But you are responsible, it is your decision, and therefore you should decide.

◻ You're trying to use the meeting to "pull a fast one" on a colleague or your boss. In other words, he or she is out of town and really responsible, but you call a meeting under guise of "an emergency" to make decisions on his or her project.

◻ You are on an ego trip and like the sound of your voice.

◻ The subject is too important to merit a meeting. That is, quick, decisive action is needed and you clearly have the necessary responsibility and authority. So step up, decide and get on with it.

◻ You've lost your case elsewhere and you are looking for a life preserver.

Create meeting protocols or norms if your group meets regularly. Consider this example[3]:

- ◻ Understand the goal of the meeting and work smart to achieve it.
- ◻ Prepare for the meeting. Review agenda, previous notes, and minutes. Understand the meeting's purpose and come ready to participate.
- ◻ Arrive promptly to avoid disrupting others.
- ◻ Bring paper and pen to take notes.
- ◻ Honor deadlines for pre and post-meeting deliverables.
- ◻ Shut off cell phones and pager ringers or set them to vibrate. If you need to answer a call or page, do it outside the meeting room.
- ◻ Be courteous and respectful of other attendees.
- ◻ Avoid sidebar discussions.
- ◻ Create a "parking lot" list during the meeting for issues that need resolution but are beyond the scope of the meeting agenda.

Prepare to deal with difficult behavior

- ◻ While careful meeting preparation is appreciated by participants and tends to bring out the best in them, some attendees may unknowingly or intentionally exhibit non-productive behavior. As a leader or facilitator of meetings, you are likely to recognize some of the following difficult behaviors and possibly appreciate some of the suggested solutions[1,4]:

TABLE 32–1. DIFFICULT BEHAVIORS IN MEETINGS AND POSSIBLE SOLUTIONS

DIFFICULT BEHAVIOR	SOLUTION(S)
Person makes clearly erroneous statement	Offer a correction. Indicate that the speaker is entitled to his or her opinion. Ask others to comment on the statement.

continued

TABLE 32–1. DIFFICULT BEHAVIORS IN MEETINGS AND POSSIBLE SOLUTIONS (CONT'D)	
DIFFICULT BEHAVIOR	**SOLUTION(S)**
Individual talks too much	Say: "Henry, I think you've made your point; let's give others an opportunity to make theirs." Say: "Heidi, our agenda is full; we must move on." Say: "Joel, that's interesting; but I think we are moving away from our agenda."
Person does not contribute	Appeal to the person's experience; say "Nancy, I understand that you have experience in this area. What is your opinion?" Appeal to the person's position; say "John, we haven't heard from the planning department. What are your concerns?"
Individual is obstinate, continues to press for a course of action even though the group is clearly opposed, at least for the time being.	Ask the person to put his or her ideas and arguments in writing for possible future reconsideration or for the record.
Person speaks, in a side conversation, to one or more individuals in low, possibly negative tone.	Pause to enable others to listen. Ask the person to repeat the comment for the benefit of the group.
Individual uses poor choice of words, erroneous terminology or pronunciation.	Help them by saying: In other words, you are saying…

Read the following related lessons

☐ Lesson 33, "Agenda Item: Good News"

☐ Lesson 34, "Minutes: Earning a Return on the Hours Invested in Meetings"

Study one or more of the following sources cited in this lesson

1. Walesh SG. Management of relationships with others. In *Engineering Your Future: The Non-Technical Side of Professional Practice in Engineering and Other Technical Fields.* 2nd ed. Reston, VA: ASCE Press; 2000.

2. Kriegel R, Brandt D. *Sacred Cows Make the Best Burgers: Paradigm-Busting Strategies for Developing Change-Ready People and Organizations.* New York: Warner Books; 1996.

3. Craumer, M. The effective meeting: A checklist for success. Harvard Management Communication Letter. March 2001.

4. Ziglar Z. *Top Performance.* New York: Berkley Books; 1986: 13–139.

Refer to the following supplemental sources

- ◻ The ten commandments of meetings. Harvard Management Communication Letter, November 1999.

- ◻ Coping with conflict. Harvard Management Communication Letter, November 2000.

- ◻ Mitchell S. Johnson W. Holding more fruitful staff meetings. *Am J Health Syst Pharm.* 1998;55:2360–2361.

Time spent on any item of the agenda
will be in inverse proportion to the sum involved.

— C. Northcote Parkinson

Agenda Item: Good News

||||||||||||||||||||||||||||||||||||||||||||||||||||||||||||||||||||||||||||||

The applause of the crowd makes the head giddy,
But the attestation of a reasonable man makes the
heart glad.

— Richard Steele

During one period in my career, I managed and led a three-department unit within an organization. Over a period of 8 years, the three department heads and I met weekly or every other week. In keeping with my nature, we operated in a systematic fashion. Agendas were issued prior to meetings, our meetings moved right along, decisions were made, and minutes were quickly distributed and posted so that all members of the unit and my "boss" could read them.

The first agenda item at each meeting was "Additional Agenda Items." This was done in recognition that, although meetings were carefully planned, something might "come up" at the last moment and require immediate attention.

The second agenda item for all meetings was "Good News." We typically quickly got to this agenda item, went around the room, and shared many specific good things that happened during the 1 to 2 weeks since the last meeting. Although we used this process for about 8 years, I cannot recall a meeting at which significant and uplifting "good news" was not reported.

Realistically, some of the "good news" was a "stretch." That is, one or more of us may have felt pressure, at a particular meeting, to dig deeply to find something "good" to report within our area of responsibility. However, the vast majority of "good news" was sincere and noteworthy. Good things were happening all around us. They warranted recognition and celebration. However, to do so the good things and the individuals and groups responsible for them had to be known.

The periodic expectation to report "good news" made me more aware of my surroundings. The upcoming need to report "good news" heightened my awareness. I suspect the department heads had a similar experience. In retrospect, that increased sensitivity was valuable in and of itself if for no other reason in that it caused me, and probably others, to listen more and talk less; to ask more questions, and make fewer statements.

Continuously learning about and celebrating "good news" is an essential element in a thriving (as opposed to surviving and dying) organization. Once our basic physical needs are met (e.g., we earn a decent income) our work satisfaction is derived largely from challenges we face and recognition we receive. Meaningful, timely recognition requires current information regarding the good things that are happening all around us and at all levels in an organization. The "good news" agenda item is a simple, effective mechanism for obtaining this information. Try it within your circle of influence.

Incidentally, you won't need a "Bad News" agenda item. That topic will take care of itself.

We are all imbued with the love of praise.

— Marcus Tullius Cicero

Suggestions for Applying Ideas

Recognize and celebrate good news through actions

- Document good news in widely distributed meeting minutes.
- Personally congratulate individuals and groups that "created" the good news by acquiring resources, completing projects, making discoveries, achieving goals or otherwise distinguishing themselves.
- Publish good news on the organization's website or in its newsletter or other periodical.

Read the following related lessons

- Lesson 21, "Caring Isn't Coddling." (The high expectations–high support philosophy advocated in this lesson will produce an abundance of good news.)
- Lessons 32 through 34 in Part 5, "Meetings"
- Lesson 38, "Our Most Important Asset"

He who praises everybody praises nobody.

— Samuel Johnson

Lesson 34

Minutes: Earning a Return on the Hours Invested in Meetings

|||||||||||||||||||||||||||||||||||||||||||||||||||||||||||||||||||||||||||||||||

A committee is a group that keeps minutes and loses hours.

— Milton Berle

I agree with Milton Berle's basic message, that is, committees, in general, and their meetings, in particular, often waste time. However, I disagree with even the suggestion that minutes are unnecessary. In fact, one of the reasons many meetings are much less effective than they could be is that they are not quickly followed by written documentation. Other reasons include poor planning, no or a weak agenda, excessive length, and rambling and diversions during the meeting.

In the absence of minutes, a meeting may, for all practical purposes, have never happened. That is, lots of talk but no action. Or, worse yet, without documentation a meeting may be remembered in as many different and conflicting ways as the number of attendees. Absent the reality check provided by minutes issued shortly after a meeting, participants tend to remember what they would like to have happened not would did happen. Given the opportunity, we tend to rewrite history in our favor, that is, edit the past so that it serves our present needs.

To avoid complications like the preceding, we should insist on minutes. These minutes should focus on decisions made and resulting action items.

Individuals who are responsible for the action items should be identified. Written minutes do not have to be long, elegant literary gems. A short, bulleted format is certainly acceptable and likely to be appreciated by recipients. My completion goal on minutes, when I prepare them or can influence their preparation, is to have minutes in hands of or on the computer screens of participants within three working days after the meeting.

The labor cost of preparing minutes is very small relative to the labor cost of preparing for and conducting the meeting (typically less than 5%). That small incremental investment of additional time is likely to be the catalyst for getting the desired return on investment of the large amount of time already invested in planning and conducting the meeting.

Suggestions for Applying Ideas

Consider recording, in real time, the key points of the discussion as a meeting progresses

- Use newsprint, transparencies, or other media readily visible to all participants.

- The chair, secretary, a facilitator or other specialty-designated person could provide this service.

- Real time minutes are particularly useful in sensitive or controversial situations where participants want to see and review what has transpired as the discussion proceeds. Everyone has the same complete record and everyone has the opportunity to question the recorder's interpretation.

- Conflicts can be resolved at the meeting as they occur instead of after the meeting when formal minutes are produced.

- The real-time minutes can be used to quickly prepare the traditional minutes for the meeting.

Allow participants to comment on meeting minutes; a group's success requires consensus on what was decided and why

- Encourage consensus by sending draft minutes to participants shortly after the meeting. Ask for review comments within an explicit time frame. Include in the transmittal email, memorandum, or letter a note that says, "If I do not hear from you within 3 days, I will assume you find the draft minutes acceptable."

- Solicit review comments from meeting participants by immediately sending the draft minutes and then asking for corrections near the beginning of the next meeting.

Read the following related lessons

- Lessons 32 through 34 in Part 5, "Meetings"
- Lesson 28, "TEAM: Together Everyone Achieves More"
- Lesson 29, "Virtual Teams"

Refer to the following supplemental sources

- Frank MO. *How to Run a Successful Meeting In Half the Time.* New York: Simon & Schuster; 1989. (Offers many specific suggestions to improve the planning and conduct of meetings. Tools and techniques range from logistics such as where to sit to ways to introduce ideas not on the prepared agenda.)

- Craumer M. The effective meeting: A checklist for success. Harvard Management Communication Letter, March 2001. (Offers suggestions on meeting follow up and follow through.)

*The meeting isn't over
until the paperwork is done.*

— Anonymous

Part 6

‖‖‖

Marketing

"Marketing" elicits intense, often negative responses from pharmacists. This is unfortunate given that, in the business sector, marketing is essential to survival. Its success depends on leadership by pharmacists, or at least an enthusiastic participation by them. Marketing is also important in government, academic, and other arenas.

Lessons in this section take a positive tact. Marketing is presented as an honorable process by which some person or organization with a need connects with someone or organization able to meet that need. Win-win outcomes occur.

A Simple Professional Services Marketing Model

||||||||||||||||||||||||||||||||||||||||||||||||||||||||||||||||||||||||||||||||||||||||||||||||||

I don't care how much you know
until I know how much you care.

— Anonymous

The word "marketing" often engenders negative reactions or connotations. The pharmacist sees images of brash, high-pressure salespeople. Pharmacists may be repulsed by the thought of "wasting" their professional education and experience doing "sales" work. Nevertheless, hopefully you will be at least receptive to the particular marketing model presented here. To the extent you learn to view marketing as earning trust and meeting customer needs, which is the essence of the model, you may conclude that not only is marketing an ethical process, but also a very satisfying and mutually beneficial one.

Marketing is a major expense for a healthcare organization—it consumes valuable hours and dollars. Therefore, the marketing effort must be carefully planned and executed. Disciplined management and enlightened leadership are required. Pharmacy departments that provide services directly to patients should undertake a continuous, proactive, positive marketing process; not a series of sporadic reactions when prescription volume or clinic visits are flat.

Marketing is not a department,
it is your business.

— Harry Beckwith

Speaker and author Stephen Covey[1] explains that the Greek philosophy for what might now be called win/win interpersonal and inter-organizational relations was based on ethos, pathos, and logos. In this model:

▢ "**Ethos** is your personal credibility, the faith people have in your integrity and competency. It's the trust that you inspire..."

▢ "**Pathos** is the empathic side—it's the feeling. It means you are in alignment with the emotional thrust of another's communication."

▢ "**Logos** is the logic, the reasoning part of the presentation."

Covey emphasizes that these three elements of win/win interpersonal and inter-organizational relations must occur in the indicated order. That is, earn trust, learn needs, and then logically follow-up.

The ethos-pathos-logos sequence offers us a positive and effective marketing model provided that the indicated sequence is followed, that is:

▢ Earn trust

▢ Learn needs

▢ Close deal

The rational tendency in interpersonal relations is to start with logos which usually lead to less than satisfactory results. Pharmacists, in particular, are inclined to proceed too quickly with and rely too heavily on logic.

Each of us, as pharmacists striving to facilitate a mutually beneficial marketing process, should first establish trust, then understand needs, and finally follow-up logically. Once trust is earned, potential partners are likely to share their needs with us in response to our questions. If there is a match, that is, if your team can be of assistance, then a logical follow-up in the form of an agreement is likely to occur.

If a match does not develop between our team and the potential partner, then we should provide assistance by referring the potential partner to another to another team. Remember that our first goal is to earn trust. Being truly helpful, by making a thoughtful referral, is one way to do that.

It takes 20 years to build a reputation,

and 5 minutes to ruin it.

If you think about that,

you'll do things differently.

— Warren Buffet

Many specific tools and techniques are available for implementing a marketing program. An effective set of tools and techniques must be selected for each of the three steps, that is, earning trust, learning needs and closing the deal. Peter Drucker, management consultant and writer, succinctly states that "The aim of marketing is to make selling superfluous." This definition underscores the idea that selling is only one small part of marketing and suggests that if marketing is done well, sales will occur naturally.

The earn trust, learn needs, and close sales marketing model is simple. However, its application requires patience and perseverance and, therefore, major absolute time and elapsed time. Elapsed time for a particular marketing effort will certainly be measured in months and more likely in years.

All pharmacists, whether in the private or public sectors, whether providing services or products, should be aware of the marketing function. Why? Because all of us ultimately help to meet patient, customer, or stakeholder needs and the essence of marketing is learning about and meeting needs. If you are employed by a healthcare consulting firm or are interested in growth of your pharmacy service, then marketing becomes a critical success factor. It should be one of your management and leadership abilities.

Suggestions for Applying Ideas

Recognize the amount of absolute and elapsed time for each of the three steps of the marketing model

▦ The first of the three steps, **earning trust**, requires by far most of the absolute and elapsed time. The second step, **learning needs,** consumes much less time. The time needed for the third step, **closing the deal**, is very small compared to the time required to earn the trust and learn the needs on which the sale is based. For example:

- For 7 years, I communicated with the president of a particular firm before discovering an opportunity to be of service. Largely as a result of the relationship that had been developed, I was selected on a sole source basis for an interesting, satisfying, and financially rewarding assignment.

- Admittedly, a 7-year trust earning–needs learning process is long. However, when marketing pharmacy and related professional services, don't expect to accomplish the personal process in weeks or even months. Select potential customers carefully and then practice patience and perseverance.

Contrast the approaches in Table 35–1 that work with approaches that do not work in the three-step earn trust–learn needs–close deal marketing model.

TABLE 35–1. MARKETING APPROACHES THAT WORK AND ONES THAT DON'T	
WHAT WORKS	**WHAT DOESN'T**
Listening to earn trust and learn needs	Talking about what we do
Building relationships	Pursuing projects
Asking questions	Pontificating
Researching, qualifying and ranking potential customers; a rifle approach	Viewing customers as being the same; a shotgun approach
Active involvement in targeted professional/business organizations	Passive membership in randomly selected professional/business organizations

TABLE 35–1. MARKETING APPROACHES THAT WORK AND ONES THAT DON'T (CONT'D)	
WHAT WORKS	**WHAT DOESN'T**
Keeping current—clinically and otherwise	Maintaining status quo
"Face time"	Mass mailings
What you see is what you get	Bait and switch
Illustrating benefits	Pushing features
Multiple level contacts with customer	Single level contact
Suggesting program and project approaches	Reacting to requests for proposals
Tailoring to customer	Boilerplating from files
Defining and meeting requirements	Talking "quality" and spewing slogans
Delivering locally while drawing globally	Attempting to do it all locally
Admitting errors and fixing them	Blaming others
Caring for existing customers—performing on their projects	Neglecting existing customers—chasing new ones
Perseverance	Instant success
Saying "thank you"	Being presumptuous

Apply the model, earn trust–learn needs–close sale, to other situations

- ◘ As noted in the essay, the model is based on a win/win approach to interpersonal and interorganizational relations.
- ◘ Successful interpersonal and interorganizational relations and accomplishments are based on earned trust and understood needs.

Just about everything we do
that is meaningful in our lives
evolves from a personal relationship

— Janet Silvester

▣ The next time we are confronted with family, neighborhood, community, or other issues, let's ask:

- Have the principal individuals earned each other's trust? If not, work on it because without trust the resolution of the issue will be, at best, fragile and highly legalistic.

- Do the principal individuals understand each others needs? If not, work on it because an acceptable resolution must try to satisfy needs.

- Can we close the deal, that is, agree to a solution or course of action? Assuming trust has been earned and needs have been learned, the answer is likely to be yes!

Read the following related lessons

▣ Lessons 36 and 37, also in the "Marketing" section of this book

Study the following source cited in this lesson

1. Covey SR. *The 7 Habits of Highly Effective People.* New York, NY: Simon & Schuster; 1990.

Refer to following supplemental sources

▣ Brown TR. Marketing pharmaceutical services. in *Handbook of Institutional Pharmacy Practice.* 4th ed. Bethesda, MD: American Society of Health System Pharmacists; 2006.

▣ Lantos PP. Marketing 101: how I got my ten largest assignments. *Journal of Management Consulting.* November 1998:38–40.

Subscribe to one or more of these e-newsletters

▣ The "LawMarketing e-Newsletter," a free e-newsletter offered by Larry Bodine, a marketing and web consultant. Provides marketing ideas, typically in the form of short pragmatic articles that are potentially useful to pharmacists even though the e-newsletter is focused on attorneys. The usefulness of this law marketing e-newsletter to pharmacists should not be surprising given the wide applicability of the basic principles underlying effective marketing. Examples of topics addressed in this e-newsletter are marketing in slow times, cross-selling, and creativity. To subscribe, go to http://www.lawmarketing.com/.

What you do with your billable time determines your current income, but what you do with your non-billable time determines your future.

— David Maister

Quickness as a Competitive Edge

||||||||||||||||||||||||||||||||||||||||||||||||||||||||||||||||||||||||||||||||||||||

In an increasingly networked economy,
it's not the big that beat the small,
but the fast that beat the slow.

— John Chambers

Several years ago, after careful research, my wife and I found just the right boat, immediately made an offer, and needed to quickly arrange financing. I called our bank, explained the situation, and asked for a financing commitment. I received the traditional "the committee will look into it" response. To my surprise, the bank officer called back in 20 minutes and indicated that they would provide financing and processing the paper work would be a formality. A pleasant quickness of service experience.

At about that time, I began using one of those "quick oil change" places. The attraction was the promise of 10-minute service. This commitment contrasted sharply with my usual "service station" which said something like "if you have your car into our place by 9:00 a.m. we should be able to have it for you by the end of the day."

At the "quick place," I could see the technician's work on the car—they exhibited enthusiasm and looked like they knew what they were doing.

They also did a lot based on the computerized list of services I received—way beyond changing the oil and filter. For example, they adjusted tire pressures and all fluid levels. This is reassuring. Finally, I don't pay any more, at least not much more, than I would at the "service station." Another example of speedier service.

I once dropped dress shirts off at the cleaners at about 9:30 a.m. The conversation went something like this: "When will these be done?" I asked. "After 3:00 p.m." the clerk said. "But on what day?" I asked. "Today!" she replied. I asked why they were trying to turn the work around more quickly. She said "We've adopted a goal of in and out on the same day to provide even better service than our competitors." Another example of faster service.

Within a week, I took a sport coat to another dry cleaners for cleaning and for minor tailoring. The conversation went something like this:

> *Clerk*: "It will be done one week from today."
>
>> Having been recently sensitized to quickness of service, I recalled that everything has always taken a week at this place.
>
> *Me*: "Why do you need a week to alter and dry clean a sport coat—surely this requires only a few hours?
>
> *Clerk*: "We have a week's backlog."
>
>> Her boss, on overhearing our conversation, came over concerned.
>
> *Boss*: "Is there a problem, sir?"
>
> *Me*: "No, I was just trying to understand why things take so long, especially compared to the other cleaner that I normally use?"
>
>> The boss assured me that everything was normal.
>
> *Boss*: "We've been backed up one week for at least 7 years."

Putting on my management hat, I suggested that, after a crash catch-up effort, they could offer one or two-day cleaning and alteration services to set themselves apart from many other similar businesses. This generated two strange looks—they just didn't get it.

And what about the healthcare industry? Here are some examples:

- ◻ Why do some task forces take months to accomplish a project when 90% of effort is expended in the last one to two meetings? Often the project could be completed in less elapsed and absolute time and at less cost.

- ◻ Why do meeting minutes always seem to come out a week or more after a meeting, if at all, especially when immediate preparation and distribution of minutes would motivate and enable meeting partici-pants to move ahead with assigned or volunteered action items?

- ◻ Why do hospital construction projects drag on for months and months, with significant periods of no activity, resulting in unneeded and unnecessary employee and patient frustration?

Given that banks, auto lubrication shops, cleaners and other businesses earn a competitive edge with efficiency, quickness could be the distinguish-ing benefit offered by healthcare organizations. Efficient service might be especially useful for clinics that provide basic health services that can easily be obtained elsewhere. Quickness without sacrificing quality and safety could differentiate these organizations from competitors. Although healthcare entities have not relied on quickness for a competitive advan-tage, speedier delivery of routine services might improve relations with patients while reducing healthcare costs.

Ingredients needed to speed up processes include self and organiza-tional discipline, identification and use of best practices, and effective use of computers and other electronic production and communication tools. Think about the advantages of quickness during the ten minutes needed for your next oil change. Some of the speedy service tactics they use may be transferable to your work environment.

Unless we hasten,
we shall be left behind.

— Lucius Annaeus Seneca

Suggestions for Applying Ideas

Apply benchmarking as a means of identifying possible ways to increase your organization's efficiency

- ▫ "Benchmarking is the continuous process of measuring products, services, and practices against the toughest competitors."[1] More simply stated, benchmarking means learning from the practices of others, whether you or they are in the public, private or volunteer sectors.

- ▫ Identify a process in your organization that needs to be done more efficiently.

- ▫ Look for organizations that excel in doing your or similar processes efficiently. Don't necessarily confine your search to competitors or even similar organizations. For example, what could your pharmacy or hospital learn about efficiency from the way Dell Computers quickly handles laptop repairs, the way Speedee Oil Change provides oil changes and related services, and the way Fedex delivers packages overnight?

- ▫ Learn as much as you can about the organizations you identify and, more specifically, their efficient processes. Possible sources of information include articles published about the processes, the organizations' websites, and asking the organizations for help.

- ▫ Integrate some of what you learn into your processes and monitor the effects on your operations.

In skating over thin ice
our safety is in our speed.

— Ralph Waldo Emerson

Read the following related lessons

- ▫ Lessons 35 and 37, also in Part 6 of this book

Study the following source cited in this lesson

1. Camp RC. *Benchmarking: The Search for Industries Best Practices that Lead to Superior Performance.* Milwaukee, WI: ASQC Quality Press; 1989.

~~~~~~~~~~~~~~~~~~~~~~~

Better three hours too soon,
Than one minute too late.

— William Shakespeare

The Chimney Sweep and the Sewer Cleaner: The Importance of Style

‖‖

Every production of genius
must be the production of enthusiasm.

— Benjamin Disraeli

Only the owner of an "older home" can fully appreciate having "everything" go wrong at once. This time "everything" included sewer and chimney problems. Tree roots had apparently once again plugged the lateral sewer. Besides a good cleaning, the fireplace chimney needed a screened cap to keep out the squirrels.

The last bushy-tailed visitor dropped onto the hearth shortly after we started a fire, sped to the dining room, and frantically jumped onto the windowsill. We opened the front door and, after taking one lap around the dining room table, the squirrel ran outside to freedom. That was enough!

The chimney sweep and the sewer cleaner were scheduled for the same day. The chimney sweep arrived, strode directly to the front door, and rang the bell. Somewhat to my wife's surprise, he was formally attired—top hat, white shirt, bow tie, and black coat with tails.

He politely introduced himself and responded to my wife's curiosity by explaining the history of chimney sweeps and, in particular, their garb.

Chimney sweeps were of the poorest class in Europe. They depended on castoffs for their clothing and often acquired the discarded formal attire of the undertakers. After excusing himself, the chimney sweep began his initial inspection of our chimney.

As the chimney sweep walked away from the front door, the sewer cleaner drove his truck into the driveway. He trudged around the house to the back door. My wife answered the doorbell and noticed that the sewer cleaner's clothing, in contrast to the chimney sweep's, was strictly functional—green work clothes and heavy boots. The sewer cleaner didn't bother to introduce himself, but instead mumbled something about the "weirdo" at the front door, and then went down into the basement to begin his work.

The chimney sweep completed his initial assessment and returned several days later with a taller ladder and special cleaning equipment. He was up and down the ladder, in and out of the house, and then back up the ladder as he went about cleaning the chimney and installing the cap.

Because our home was on a busy street, the chimney sweep attracted considerable attention and many passing motorists sounded their horns. During one of his trips into the house, the chimney sweep explained that the proper response to greetings from the passers-by was a tip of the hat and bow from his position at the top of the ladder. However, he was frustrated because the traffic was so heavy and the beeping so persistent that he simply could not take the time to give the traditional tip of the hat and bow. Therefore, he compromised and simply waved. After completing his work, the chimney sweep presented his bill, and politely said good-bye.

Chimney work is probably no more or no less important than sewer work. In terms of desirability and prestige, both trades would probably rank low. And yet, there was something special about the way our chimney was cleaned compared to the way our sewer was unplugged. I suspect that the cheery, enthusiastic chimney sweep felt better about cleaning the chimney than did the glum sewer cleaner about unplugging the sewer. While both the chimney sweep and the sewer cleaner provided valuable services to us, the chimney sweep did it in such a way so as to bring a bit of cheer to us and to the many passersby.

This story illustrates an important point. Although the work we do is important, the manner in which we do it significantly affects the way our efforts are received and appreciated by others. Think of your favorite restaurant, hardware store, or hair stylist. While the quality and price of products or services help to define "favorite," I suspect that the attitude of employees combined with the physical setting enters into the equation.

The same style principle applies to pharmacists. More specifically, style enhances marketing like frosting on a cake or the bow on a package. As we seek new customers, and strive to improve service to existing ones, let's explicitly include style in the effort. Exude enthusiasm, be polite, listen carefully, speak clearly, explain thoughtfully, assist positively, dress appropriately, walk tall, and smile!

Enthusiasts soon understand each other.

— Washington Irving

Suggestions for Applying Ideas

Assess the style of your organization, or the portion for which you are responsible

- ⬚ Try to imagine you are a patient, customer, or other stakeholder. Forget what you know about your workplace and the people who work there.

  - "Call yourself up," as suggested by Robert Townsend,[1] the former CEO of the Avis rental car company. Put yourself in the customer's shoes and call your organization. What is your perception? If it's negative, how could it be fixed?

  - Approach and enter your building. Do the external and internal physical environment speak of what you do and how you do it? Does the setting convey the importance of your organization's work and the pride you take in it? Or is it generic and bland?

- ⬚ Better yet, ask a friend, who knows little about your organization, to do the preceding. Eliminate the need to imagine you are an outsider.

⬛ Consider this anecdote. While I was serving as a faculty member, a prospective student and her mother met with me as part of a visit to our campus. They had already visited at least one other campus. Mother immediately said something like, "I really like your school compared to the one we visited yesterday." Obviously, I asked why. Her answer: The entrance to our building was neat and clean. Of course faculty, curricula, and laboratories are important, but so is the style of the place.

More often than not,
things and people are as they appear.

— Malcolm Forbes

Read the following related lessons

⬛ Lessons 35 and 36, also in Part 6 of this book

Study the following source cited in this lesson

1. Townsend R. *Up The Organization: How to Stop Corporations from Stifling People and Strangling Profits.* New York: Alfred A. Knopf; 1970.

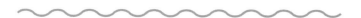

Promotion awaits the employee who radiates cheerfulness,
not the employee who spreads gloom and dissatisfaction.

— B.C. Forbes

Part 7

||||||||||||||||||||||||||||||||||||||||||||||||||||||||||||||||||||||||||||||||

Building Mutually Beneficial Employee-Employer Partnerships

Question for employers: What goes down the elevator and out the door every day? Answer: Your most important "asset." Your personnel.

Question for employees: As you go down the elevator and out the door, what determines whether or not you look forward to returning tomorrow? Answer: Probably a mixture of tangible and intangible factors that define the success and significance of your work.

The old employer-employee contract, under which the former toils faithfully and the latter guarantees a job, is largely gone. In its place is a more sophisticated, challenging and improved model under which both parties seek deep and broad benefits and each is free to discontinue the relationship if its productivity declines.

Employers need to examine their recruitment and retention process to recognize today's realities. Similarly, prospective employees should carefully conduct their job searches. Lessons in this section offer advice to both employees and employers.

Our Most Important Asset

|||||||||||||||||||||||||||||||||||||||||||||||||||||||||||||||||||||||||||||||||||||||

Hire the best.
Pay them fairly.
Communicate frequently.
Provide challenges and rewards.
Believe in them.
Get out of their way and
they'll knock your socks off.

— Mary Ann Allison

I don't know what our second most valuable resource is, but it doesn't matter. With competent, creative and conscientious people, our organizations can do almost anything. Without such people, regardless of what other resources we may have, we will struggle simply to survive. So how do we retain this valuable asset, the skilled human resource, which is so expensive to recruit in the first place, and prevent them from leaving for oftentimes perceived better alternatives?

As the recent pharmacy staffing survey indicated, the continued increase in the vacancy rates in the presence of no changes in the relatively high turnover rates means that pharmacy managers must increasingly focus on the most important asset, the human resource.[1] In this era of pharmacy workforce shortages, highly effective and productive personnel are difficult to find. This scarcity has caused more employees to seek better opportunities in terms of financial rewards and/or job satisfaction.

In my view, the most important factor in the effective retention and utilization of personnel is creating and building long lasting relationships. It is natural to focus on personnel as individuals who perform work and the role of managers or leaders is to develop skills to produce high quality work. This approach is described by many as a management by objectives approach. Though this approach is appropriate in achieving departmental objectives, recognize that the most motivated and productive members of the team are those who have strong relationships with others including those for whom they work. When personnel realize that the leader genuinely cares and is interested in the success of their personal and professional life, they form a covenant of trust and as a result they are motivated to be a productive member of the team. Below are the basic elements of a caring relationship provided by Paul Abramowitz in his publication on nurturing relationships.[2]

- ◻ Paying attention through active listening.
- ◻ Displaying understanding by mirroring ideas.
- ◻ Giving others credit for their ideas.
- ◻ Welcoming feedback and an honest exchange of information, without threat of punishment
- ◻ Staying accessible.
- ◻ Being polite and courteous in everyday interactions.
- ◻ Expressing gratitude for hard work.
- ◻ Seeking to discover and nurture the unique skills that each person brings to the workplace.
- ◻ Showing a willingness to trust
- ◻ Sharing with and opening up to others.

All of the above elements collectively work together to create an environment of trust and encourages motivation to perform better. Exercising the elements is a responsibility of the leader and as such he or she should be held accountable to those standards.

It begins with a natural feeling that one wants to serve, to serve first.
Then conscious choice brings one to aspire to lead …
The difference manifests itself in the care taken by the servant – first to make sure other people's highest priority needs are being served.

— Robert K. Greenleaf

Enlightened education and training (E&T) is also a part of the answer to effective utilization and retention of personnel resources for individual and the organizational benefit. Consider these suggestions:

- Audit your E&T efforts. Consult with a pharmacy management expert to help you take a fresh look at how you spend resources. Are you cost-effectively investing resources (time and dollars) so that they yield an attractive return on investment (ROI) by meeting your organization's clinical and financial outcomes, and other needs? Or, is E&T just another expense and poorly managed at that?

- Partner with your personnel on designing and developing the E&T programs. Both you and they should invest time and dollars for maximum ROI.

- Experiment with various teaching and learning mechanisms including rapidly emerging distance-learning technologies such as web-based training. Younger personnel, in particular, are likely to embrace these. One-on-one education sessions with experts can also yield high retention rates as they can be tailored and customized to meet individual needs.

- Leverage your E&T investments. For example, require some form of reporting, sharing, or action from each person who participates in any learning activity.

▪ Implement coaching (easy) or mentoring (difficult) programs as a proactive way for senior personnel to share knowledge with junior personnel.

Besides E&T, other enlightened means are available to retain high quality personnel, that is, to cultivate our most important assets. One is to recognize individual and group technical and non-technical achievements. We work for different reasons but most of us value timely and sincere private and public recognition. Most pharmacist or pharmacy personnel enjoy working in a challenging environment that includes a high degree of direct patient contact. Make this or other desired but feasible environments available to the personnel. Following are some of the other ways to retain your most valuable asset, as described by Leigh Branham in his book *Keeping the People Who Keep You in Business*[3]:

1. Inspire a commitment to a clear vision and definite objectives
2. Redesign the job itself to make it more rewarding
3. Define the results you expect and the talent you need
4. Hire and promote managers who have the talent to manage people
5. Creatively expand your talent pool
6. Communicate how their work is vital to the organization's success
7. Challenge early and often
8. Train managers in career coaching and expect them to do it
9. Know when to keep and when to let go
10. Have more fun!

Our most important assets go down the elevator or out the door everyday. Managers and leaders are best positioned to fix this problem. Leaders and managers should determine future service needs, build lasting relationships, and use E&T and other means to recruit, retain and strengthen the best and brightest personnel to meet those needs. Established guidelines that pertain to pharmacy practice are available in the literature to assist with planning.[4] It is in the best interest of the manager or leader to build and develop a strong team of caring and high achieving individuals. This approach practices good stewardship while helping the bottom line.

Pursuit of individual independence is rapidly coming to a close as we move towards more interdependence.

— David A. Zilz

Suggestions for Applying Ideas

Assess the management style of the leaders of the pharmacy department. Are the leaders focused on a no-nonsense management by objective approach or do they lead the department by building relationships with key individuals to achieve departmental objectives?

- ▢ Does your organization develop standards of behavior that pertain to building relationships amongst personnel and between personnel and leadership?

- ▢ Discuss at a management team meeting how the aforementioned basic elements of relationship building can be employed within your setting to motivate personnel and build creativity within the team.

- ▢ Hold managers and leaders accountable for making relationship building a top priority.

- ▢ Schedule management rounds and make personal visits to each departmental area at least once per month. Prepare notes on feedback, issues, concerns, etc. Utilize notes at management team meetings to identify resolutions and associated priorities. Execute the planned action steps to create the desired environment

Influence your organization's culture by empowering and developing its personnel, particularly if you are in a position to do so

◘ Contemplate the experience and observations of John Mole, who wrote *Management Mole: Lessons from Office Life,*[5]

- John Mole, an educated and experienced manager, quit his management position and went underground for two years as a "mole."

- During that time, he had temporary jobs in 11 organizations; jobs he obtained without revealing his education and business background.

- His disturbing observations, as presented in the book, are as follows:

  - The majority of junior-level staff he encountered wanted to learn, work, contribute, and succeed.

  - Unfortunately, much of that potential was wasted because of poor management and leadership. Orientation, education, and training were virtually non-existent. As a result, the "blind lead the blind."

◘ Is your organization tapping and enabling its people resources? Or are you letting them flounder?

*Making sure that everyone in the organization
knows exactly what his job is
and what its purpose is
and how it fits in—
and how you know you are doing well—
is an arduous and never ending process,
but it's the single most important element in managing people*

— John Mole

Use "people assets" to help your organization rise to greatness

◘ Management researcher Jim Collins in his book *Good to Great*[6] observes that good companies rise to greatness because of their people. Some other observations:

☐ "People are not your most important asset. The right people are." This statement supports and gives added emphasis to the theme of this lesson's essay.

☐ Individuals who led companies that ascended from good to great almost all shared two traits: personal humility and professional will. "Their ambition is first and foremost for the institution, not themselves." So much for charisma?

☐ The most effective leaders "look out the window to apportion credit. At the same time, they look in the mirror to apportion responsibility."

☐ Somewhat surprisingly, the path from good to great did not typically begin with a vision and strategy. It did not start with deciding "where to drive the bus." Instead, successful leaders "first got the right people on the bus and the wrong people off the bus" and then figured where to drive it. Stated differently, begin with "who," then address the "what."

☐ "Put your best people in your biggest opportunities, not your biggest problems." This advice counters the tendency to invest the knowledge, skills and attitudes of our star personnel in fixing big messes created by others.

☐ Don't waste time and energy trying to motivate people. Instead invest time and energy in finding and hiring motivated people and work hard to support them, to not de-motivate them.

The purpose of bureaucracy is to
compensate for incompetence and lack of discipline—
a problem that largely goes away
if you have right people in the first place.

— Jim Collins

Read the following related lessons

☐ Lesson 28, "TEAM: Together Everyone Achieves More

☐ Lessons 39 through 41, also in Part 7 of this book

Study one or more of the following sources cited in this lesson

1. Pedersen CA, Schneider PJ, Scheckelhoff DJ. ASHP national survey of pharmacy practice in hospital settings: dispensing and administration—2005. *Am J Health Syst Pharm.* 2006; 63:327–345.

2. Abramowitz PW. Nurturing relationships: an essential ingredient of leadership. *Am J Health-Syst Pharm.* 2001;58:479–484.

3. Branham FL. *Keeping the People Who Keep You in Business.* 1st ed. New York: Amazon; 2001.

4. American Society of Health-System Pharmacists. ASHP guidelines on the recruitment, selection, and retention of pharmacy personnel. *Am J Health-Syst Pharm.* 2003;60:587–593.

5. Mole J. *Management Mole: Lessons from Office Life.* London: Bantam Press; 1998.

6. Collins J. *Good to Great: Why Some Companies Make the Leap and Others Don't.* New York: Harper Business; 2001.

Interviewing So Who You Get Is Who You Want

|||||||||||||||||||||||||||||||||||||||||||||||||||||||||||||||||||||||||||||||||||||

*Remember: A's hire A's
and B's hire C's.*

— Donald Rumsfeld

The success of the Pharmacy Department depends on the quality of the team members or people who make up the department. Selection of appropriate individuals for the right position is directly correlated with employee satisfaction and the subsequent success of the organization. The one person who loses most when the right person is not selected for a particular job is the manager or leader of the department. Hence, managers or leaders must take responsibility and accountability for building a successful team by establishing and maintaining an effective recruitment process.

I recently had an opportunity to interview several candidates for a supervisor position. This position would be responsible for managing approximately 20 pharmacists and an equal number of technicians. As part of a routine interview, I studied the candidate's resume and, over lunch, asked this candidate many questions. For example, I inquired about positions he had held, the types of projects he worked on, and his accomplishments. To me, he looked great on paper and in person! He was hired. To my and my team's dismay, the new supervisor quickly and clearly demonstrated his inability to manage multiple tasks with the necessary quickness and level of attention to detail. He realized this mismatch and resigned within months.

This interviewing experience crystallized for me the importance of a carefully designed interview and selection process. Finding individuals whose manager and leader profile match the culture and needs of your organization is a challenge. Therefore, a thorough and systematic interview process is needed. As nicely stated by oil business executive J. Paul Getty, "the employer generally gets the employees he deserves." The process, which should begin with careful study of the resumes and other submittals and reference checks, might include all or most of the following five steps:

1. Define, in writing, the knowledge, skills, and attitudes needed for the position. Call these the criteria. When defining the criteria the manager must also review the departmental goals and objectives and the role of the candidate in accomplishing these goals. Discuss the criteria with individuals who would be working with and/or directly report to the candidate. This step, assuming it is a team effort, may reveal unexpected, widely divergent views on "what we are looking for." If so, get consensus before proceeding. The object of the interview is to determine the degree to which a candidate satisfies the criteria.

2. Arrange, to the extent feasible, for the candidate to explicitly demonstrate compatibility with the criteria during the interview visit. Examples of criteria that can be demonstrated during an interview are writing, speaking, and problem assessment and solution.

3. Consider reviewing examples of work products as a way of assessing a candidate's ability to meet some knowledge, skills and attitudes criteria. Assume a criterion is effective project management skills. Ask the candidate to bring and display some examples of projects led or managed. Request that the candidate discuss challenges experienced and how they were overcome or resolved.

4. Use what is sometimes called behavioral interviewing for those criteria not amenable to explicit demonstration or "show and tell"

during the interview. With this approach, the candidate is asked to relate actual personal, and hopefully revealing, experiences that illustrate desired attributes. Assuming the responses honestly portray his or her behavior, this technique is based on the premise that recent behavior is the best predictor of near future behavior.

5. Recognize that positive interpersonal "chemistry" is an important, but often-unstated criterion, in personnel selection. Accordingly, a variety of independently derived views of the candidate's potential team members and colleagues are desired. Schedule private, one-on-one and group discussions between the candidate and representative members of your organization's staff. Encourage both parties to be open and direct. Ask each involved staff member to brief the leader of the interview effort in person and/or in writing, shortly after the discussion. Evaluation forms can be developed in advance to assist team members in focusing the interview discussion and questions pertaining to the criteria.

A thorough interviewing process will put you in an excellent position to answer a very important question: Which candidate is most likely to enter into a mutually beneficial relationship with our organization? You and others will now know. You have done your homework.

~~~~~~~~~~~~~~~~~~~~~~

*It's much less expensive
to recruit from the top of the barrel
by paying top wages.*

— Robert Townsend

Suggestions for Applying Ideas

To the extent feasible, have candidates demonstrate compatibility with the position criteria during the interview visit

▢ If writing ability is one criterion for a position, obtain a sample of the candidate's writing during the interview, preferably near the end of the on-site visit. Invite the candidate to write about ways in which personal experience and aspirations are in sync with the available position and the organization's mission. Provide a quiet spot, paper or computer, and allot about one-half hour. A good to excellent writer will shine on this essay "test."

▢ If speaking is critical, request that the candidate make a presentation or conduct a workshop on a topic related to the available position. Include this requirement in the interview invitation, and indicate the allotted time. Your candidate could describe a completed project; or demonstrate knowledge of contemporary pharmacy practice or health-systems; or teach participants, in an interactive workshop mode, how to be a successful preceptor or mentor.

▢ If the ability to plan or manage complex projects is critical for the position, give the candidate an actual or hypothetical situation and about one-half hour of quiet time. Ask him or her to list questions as part of the planning process that should be answered by the organization's personnel before beginning the project.

There is something that is much more scarce,
something rarer than ability.
It is the ability to recognize ability.

— Robert Half

Use behavioral interviewing

▢ For example, assume that persistence is a desired quality. Ask the interviewee to cite a personal experience that demonstrated persistence.

▢ You can easily imagine using this behavioral approach to check out other potentially desirable qualities such as creativity, leadership, and teamwork.

▫ The retrospective, reality-based, behavioral approach contrasts sharply with the prospective, hypothetical approach. An illustration of the latter is "What would you do to encourage out-of-the-box thinking on your team?" An example of the former or behavioral approach is "Give me an example of how you encouraged out-of-the-box thinking on your team?" Slightly different wording, markedly different question.

▫ Concrete, historic examples reveal much more than hypothetical projections. Knowing what someone did do is much more valuable than what someone says they would do.

Discern the potential of candidates by looking for the following leadership traits[1,2]:

▫ Drive

▫ Motivation

▫ Integrity

▫ Self-confidence

▫ Intelligence

▫ Knowledge

Be mindful of candidates' attitudes;
they are as important as skills and experience,
and harder to change.

— Mel Hensey

Institute programs in the organization that are known to attract high quality personnel, in addition to meeting other purposes

▫ A progressive education and training program will tend to attract "top" personnel. High quality professionals want to maintain their competence and, therefore, tend to join and remain in organizations that value and support education and training.[3]

▢ The organization's ability to participate in internship, clerkship, and residency training is another way to attract "top" candidates. When given a choice, the top students and new graduates tend to choose the more challenging experiences such as intensive rotations or advanced or specialty residency training. Employers get a very close look at the performance of the students and/or residents and can evaluate them for possible full-time employment, without any obligation to pursue them. Similarly, potential candidates undergoing training (again without any obligation for future employment) have an opportunity to assess the employer. As a result, better employer-employee matches occur. This directly correlates with a high retention rate.

Avoid these hiring pitfalls based largely on ideas offered by psychologist Lester L. Tobias[4]:

▢ "Hiring expediently under the pressure of time. That's the 'buy now, pay later' approach."

▢ "Resorting to hiring the 'best of the batch' out of desperation."

▢ Compromising standards by arguing "don't some of us have to be Indians and not chiefs?"

▢ Hiring cast-offs of superb organizations or the stars of mediocre organizations.

▢ Not liking what is seen but "hiring with the hope the person will change" once they come on board. Is the unmotivated person likely to become motivated? Is the underachiever likely to achieve? Is the narrowly focused individual likely to expand his or her horizon? I doubt it.

▢ Failing to determine if the candidate has the necessary knowledge and skills.

▢ Weighing knowledge and skills too much relative to attitude.

▢ Hiring without carefully checking credentials and prior performance.

▢ Relying too much on answers to prospective, hypothetical questions and too little on responses to the retrospective, behavioral questions.

- "Ignoring your personal feelings or gut reactions."
- Insisting on cloning yourself.

Lastly, realize that the interview process is only a snapshot of a moment in time when often both the employer and employee may be under unusual circumstances to make personnel changes. The interview day is often "dressed-up" in that, the employer's desire to be a good host in order to recruit or fill a long-standing open position and the candidate's urgency to vacate from a potentially unfulfilling (incompatible) position. Each party may unconsciously attempt to please one another unnecessarily. This is a common occurrence, especially in the current state of our profession experiencing severe shortages in the workforce and demanding responsibilities of the positions. Therefore, it is particularly important for the manager to maintain focus on the predetermined criteria in light of the challenging circumstances. As documented in a recent popular publication, given the type of organization and its mission, getting the wrong personnel "off the bus" can be challenging.[5] Early assessment mechanisms, such as a well-designed interview process, can be important to avoid hiring mistakes.

Read the following related lessons

- Lessons 38 and 41, also in Part 7 of this book

Study one or more of the following sources cited in this lesson

1. Kirkpatrick SA, Locke EA. Leadership: do traits matter? *Academy of Management Executives.* May 1991:48–60.

2. Donnelly JH, Gibson JL, Ivancevich JM. *Fundamentals of Management.* 9th ed. Chicago, IL: Irwin; 1995:377–411.

3. American Society of Health-System Pharmacists. ASHP guidelines on recruitment, selection, and retention of Pharmacy Personnel. *Am J Health-System Pharm.* 2003;60:587–593.

4. The listed pitfalls are based, in part, on Tobias, L.L. Hiring for excellence. *Industry Week.* April 20, 1987: 71.

5. Collins J. *Good to Great*. New York: HarperCollins Publishers Inc; 2001.

If you want a track team to win the high jump,
you find one person who can jump seven feet,
not seven people who can jump one foot.

— Paul Dickson

Lesson 40

Eagles and Turkeys

||||||||||||||||||||||||||||||||||||||||||||||||||||||||||||||||||||||||||||||||||||||||

Walk with wise men
and you'll be wise.
But keep company with fools
and you'll suffer for it.

— Proverbs 13:20, The Bible, An American Translation

If we want to fly like eagles, we cannot get our wings from turkeys. The aspiring manger and leader in us must have regular contact with individuals who are accomplished in managing and leading—the eagles. However, we can learn what not to do from the latter—the turkeys.

Think of members of the pharmacy community, or probably any community, as being represented by a normal distribution. Eagles are found at the extreme right end. The vast majority of us occupy most of the area under the curve. We are a decent, hardworking bunch. The turkeys, that is, the whiners, cynics, grumblers, complainers, talkers, incompetents, and malcontents, occupy the extreme left end of the distribution.

Bosses, co-workers, and customers influence our attitude toward the pharmacy profession, affect the knowledge and skills we acquire, and place us in various networks. Unless you are an unusually independent, self-disciplined person, your people environment will shape you. Therefore, strive to align at least some of that people environment with your desired roles and goals. Stated differently, try to spend some time with eagles over at the extreme right end of the distribution.

I do not apologize for advising you to seek contact with accomplished individuals. In spite of all of this world's problems, its population includes a small minority of conscientious, competent, and communicative managers and leaders—visionaries who act with honesty and integrity, set and achieve goals, exhibit courage, accommodate ambiguity and chaos, and are innovative and creative. Celebrate their presence and associate with and learn from them.

> Depend on no man, on no friend
> but him who can depend on himself.
> He only who acts conscientiously toward himself,
> will act so toward others.
>
> — Johann Kaspar Lavater

Sure, we can learn about managing and leading through formal education, by reading the literature and as a result of our mistakes. However, our learning will be accelerated by frequent working contact with individuals who possess the knowledge, skills and attitudes we desire.

Just as real eagles (i.e., the majestic birds) are out there but hard to find, so is the case with those accomplished in managing and leading. How do we find these people? Three suggestions:

- Look within all types of organizations and groups such as hospitals, health systems, colleges of pharmacy, government entities, volunteer groups, service clubs, business and professional societies, and neighborhood associations. Do not limit your search to pharmacy groups.

- Scan these organizations and groups vertically. Appreciate that the most accomplished managers may be closer to the top of the organizations and groups, and hold management titles.

◻ Recognize that some of the more accomplished leaders—that is, those who influence primarily by their presence rather than positions—may not be immediately identified. They tend to eschew titles, trappings and outward signs. Instead, they are widely known by their positive, supportive influences on others. So simply ask the "others" who they look up to. If leadership is present, you will immediately find the source.

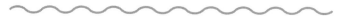

Thus you will know them by their fruits.

— Matthew 7:20, The Bible, RSV

Having found one or more of those individuals who exhibit exemplary managing and leading ability, seek ways to have meaningful contact with them. For example, depending on the situation:

◻ Volunteer to serve on their task force.

◻ Request a transfer to their department.

◻ Join their professional society.

◻ Seek their advice.

Once you've found and connected with an individual who excels in managing and leading, your real work begins. Earn his or her trust by working diligently and smart while demonstrating honesty, integrity and competence. Then you will be amazed at what you, your new teacher, and others accomplish.

Keep away from people who try to belittle your ambitions.
Small people always do that,
but the really great make you feel that you, too,
can become great.

— Mark Twain

Suggestions for Applying Ideas

Carefully choose your co-workers and your boss, especially in the early, more formative part of your career

◘ Consider employment factors such as the following: geographic location, compensation, likely projects and functions, available computer and other equipment and style/condition of office and/or work area.

◘ However, if you have high managing and leading aspirations, carefully choose your co-workers and your bosses; they are the most important factors early in your career.

*We've never succeeded
in making a good deal
with a bad person.*

— Warren Buffet

As you seek people with whom you can develop mutual trust, be alert to these six character flaws[1]

◘ People who rarely do what they say they will do.

◘ People who push their work onto you.

◘ People who are late and don't apologize.

◘ People who tell you "I'm too busy."

◘ People who reject your ideas out-of-hand.

◘ People who won't let you off the hook.

In other words, "Place high value on trust, but don't be trusting too soon."

~~~~~~~~~~~~~~~~~~~~~~

Avoid the reeking herd,
shun the polluted flock
live like the stoic bird
the eagle on the rock.

— Elinor Wylie

Read the following related lessons

◫ Lesson 1, "Leading, Managing, and Producing"

◫ Lesson 38, 39, and 41, also in Part 7 of this book

Study the following source cited in the text

1. McCormack MH. *Staying Street Smart in the Internet Age.* New York: Viking Penguin, 2000.

~~~~~~~~~~~~~~~~~~~~~~

Choose your friends
like thy books,
few but choice.

— Elbert Hubbard

KSA (Knowledge, Skills, and Attitudes)

Often our attitude is the only difference between our success and failure.

— Abraham Lincoln

Valuable knowledge and skills and positive attitudes; we want all three in the people we work with. By knowledge, I mean essentially unchanging, highly valued, and widely applicable fundamentals usually acquired through formal education. Examples are understanding pharmacy practice, drug therapy and the fundamentals of project management.

Skill refers to that which is typically acquired by training and experience, and while valued is often of transient value. Examples are ability to use a particular pharmacy computer system or dosage calculator.

Attitudes, the third desired attribute, are the ways in which one thinks or feels in response to a fact or situation. Our attitudes reflect how we "see" the world about us, not visually, but in terms of perceiving, interpreting and approaching. Leadership author John C. Maxwell says "your behavior follows your attitude. The two cannot be separated.[1]" Concentration camp survivor Viktor Frankl observed, "God chooses what we go through. We choose how we go through it."

Attitudes drive behavior. We are subjected to and experience the behavior of others and vice versa. In my view, examples of positive attitudes are commitment, curiosity, high expectations for self and others, optimism, persistence, sensitivity, and thoroughness. Negative attitudes include vacillation, pessimism, crudeness, reactiveness, and low expectations.

Positive attitudes are contagious and can have productive, catalytic, and synergistic effects within the professional practice of pharmacy. These attitudes accelerate careers and are essential to those who aspire to lead.

Great efforts spring
naturally from great attitude.

— Pat Riley

Negative attitudes tend to limit an individual's ability to fully appreciate the potential application of what they know, that is, their knowledge and skills. These undesirable attitudes hamper the individual's effectiveness within the typically complex workgroup and stakeholder environments. Negative attitudes tend to isolate an individual, stifle his or her efforts, agitate others, and deny everyone the full benefit of the individual's knowledge and skills.

Occasionally I am asked or hear a question like this: How can we motivate employees; how can we create positive attitudes within them? Most such questions are, in effect, admissions that we have hired people with poor to lousy attitudes.

Such questions prompt the question: Why did you hire these people? I am sure there are understandable answers such as we were in a jam and needed someone quickly or we were fooled by the candidate. But these kinds of answers rarely justify bringing bad attitudes into an organization. The short term benefit is not worth the long term cost.

Ideally, let's recruit and hire individuals with the requisite knowledge and skills plus positive attitudes. Second best is to hire for attitude and then help the individual further develop their knowledge and skills. Never hire someone with a poor to lousy attitude, regardless of their knowledge and skills.

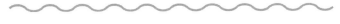

Hire attitude and train for skill.
The most talented person will destroy
a business if there is an attitude problem,
and fellow employees are the first to know it.

— Bruce Flohr

Given the age of personnel we hire, thinking we can change their attitude after they join our organization is not realistic. We are ill-equipped to be in the attitude change business, although we can and should partner with our personnel in the education and training arena. Leave basic attitude development to parents, the community, and K through 12 teachers and possibly college professors.

Some suggestions for assessing the attitudes of job candidates for a position:

1. Define, in writing, the knowledge, skills and attitudes—especially attitudes—needed for the position and arrive at some form of consensus within the department.

2. Contact references and ask them attitude questions.

3. Use behavioral interviewing focused on the desired attitudes. Repeatedly ask a candidate to share actual personal, and hopefully revealing, experiences that reveal attitudes. For example: "Tell me about a time you experienced a major setback and what you did about it." Behavioral interviewing is based on the premise that recent behavior is the best predictor of near future behavior. (Note: Behavioral interviewing contrasts with hypothetical situation interviewing in which the candidate is asked what he or she would do in a hypothetical situation—not what he or she did in an actual situation. Behavioral interviewing is retrospective, based on fact, while hypothetical interviewing is prospective and based on conjecture.)

4. Arrange, to the extent feasible, for the candidate to explicitly demonstrate, during the interview visit, desired knowledge and skill sets. For example, if speaking is an important criterion, ask the candidate to give a presentation on a project they completed. Search for basic attitudes during the presentation and subsequent question and answer period.

As we strive to improve our organizations, forget about motivating people. Instead, don't un-motivate the motivated individuals. And, the principal message of this lesson: hire motivated personnel, support them, and get out of the way. W.W. Ziege put it this way: "Nothing can stop the [person] with the right mental attitude from achieving [his/her] goal; nothing on earth can help the [person] with the wrong mental attitude."

Suggestions for Applying Ideas

Incorporate behavioral interview questions into your interviewing technique[2]

Tell me about a time when you . . .

1. Worked effectively under pressure.
2. Handled a difficult situation with a co-worker.
3. Were creative in solving a problem.
4. Missed an obvious solution to a problem.
5. Were unable to complete a project on time.
6. Persuaded team members to do things your way.
7. Wrote a report that was well received.
8. Anticipated potential problems and developed preventive measures.
9. Had to make an important decision with limited facts.
10. Were forced to make an unpopular decision.
11. Had to adapt to a difficult situation.
12. Were tolerant of an opinion that was different from yours.

13. Were disappointed in your behavior.

14. Used your political savvy to push a program through that you really believed in.

15. Had to deal with an irate customer.

16. Delegated a project effectively.

17. Surmounted a major obstacle.

18. Set your sights too high (or too low).

19. Prioritized the elements of a complicated project.

20. Got bogged down in the details of a project.

21. Lost (or won) an important contract.

22. Made a bad decision.

23. Had to fire a friend.

24. Hired (or fired) the wrong person.

25. Turned down a good job.

Read the following related lessons

- Lesson 38 and 39, also in Part 7 of this book

Study one or more of the following sources cited in this lesson

1. Maxwell JC. *Thinking for a Change.* New York: Warner Business Books; 2003.

2. Hirsch A. *Job Search and Career Checklists: 101 Proven Time-Saving Checklists to Organize and Plan Your Career Search.* Indianapolis, IN: JIST Works; 2005.

   Note: This lesson is based, in part on ideas presented in the report Civil Engineering Body of Knowledge for the 21st Century published by the American Society of Civil Engineers in 2004.

Study one or more of the following supplemental sources

▫ Foster C, Goodkin L. Employment selection in healthcare: The case for structured interviewing. *Health Care Management Review.* 1998;23(1):46–51.

▫ Holdford DA. Human Resources Management Functions. In: Desselle SP, Zgarrick DP. Eds. *Pharmacy Management: Essentials for All Practice Settings.* New York: McGraw-Hill. 2005:171–183.

▫ Behavioral Interviews: Use Behavioral Interviewing to Select the Best. Susan M. Heathfield. Available at: http:// humanresources.about.com/od/interviewing/a/behavior_interv.htm Accessed April 29, 2007.

▫ Build individual accountability. In: Studer Q, ed. *Hardwiring Excellence.* Gulf Breeze, FL: Fire Starter Publishing; 2003: 167–187.

▫ Skills, Knowledge, and Talents. In: Buckingham M, Coffman C, eds. *First, Break All the Rules.* New York, NY: Simon & Schuster; 1999: 83–92.

Any fact facing us is not as important as our attitude toward it, for that determines our success or failure.

— Norman Vincent Peale

Part 8

||||||||||||||||||||||||||||||||||||||||||||||||||||||||||||||||||||||||||||||||||||||||||||

The Broad View

Unlike all the preceding sections of this book, which tend to be pragmatic, this section is somewhat philosophical. By that I mean the enclosed essays explore concepts and values related to the pharmacy profession. Topics discussed include the challenge of effecting change, giving back to our profession and community, the different professional cultures and looking ahead at our individual futures and the future of the profession.

AH HA! A Process for Effecting Change

|||||||||||||||||||||||||||||||||||||||||||||||||||||||||||||||||||||||||||||||

*Faced with the choice between changing one's mind
and proving that there is no need to do so,
almost everybody gets busy on the proof.*

— John Kenneth Galbraith

Implementing a change in the medication process, such as a well-established medication safety initiative like requiring all medication orders written by prescribers to be legible, to include the date and time of the order and to not contain unsafe abbreviations can be challenging. The change process typically includes revision of policies, development of educational materials and presentations to those impacted by the change. Many prescribers comply after learning of the change and the rationale for it, but there are always a significant number that are slow to change or oppose it. Why is it that we often react negatively to the possibility of change? Why are we so willing to invest heavily in justifying the status quo?

Our frequent knee jerk resistance to change is usually not, in my view, based on satisfaction with current conditions. Intellectually, we know that just about anything could be improved. Our resistance is more likely to be emotional; we fear giving up that which is known, familiar, and comfortable in exchange for the possibility, but not certainty, of improvement. It's not so much the proposed improvement that frightens us but rather the transition from here to there, the letting go of that which is familiar before being able to grab onto that which could be better.

Niccolo Machiavelli, the Italian politician and writer, forcefully characterized the intensity of negative reactions to possible change and the challenge of effecting substantive change: "There is nothing more difficult to plan, more doubtful of success, nor more dangerous to manage than the creation of a new system. For the initiator has the enmity of all who would profit by the preservation of the old institutions and merely lukewarm defenders in those who would gain by the new one." [1]

Doing Our Homework: Why Do We Do What We Do?

Prior to starting the change process, we must do our homework. For example, ask "why do we do it the way we do it?" Maybe the original rationale no longer applies. The following story emphasizes the importance of determining the origin of the current system.

Proper orientation and training of our new staff is a major priority of our department to assure that these individuals are competent and confident. The training plan is documented in a department policy and procedure and each new employee completes a checklist specifically designed for their position. There are a number of required competencies, including cultural, safety, age-specific, and regulatory compliance. Training and testing is accomplished via both live and computer-based presentations with post-tests. After receiving several comments that orientation was inefficient and repetitive, we investigated and learned that much of the material in the live presentations had been added to the computer-based training provided by the training department. For more than a year we had been requiring this duplicative training. After learning of the duplication, we discontinued the live training.

All truth goes through three stages.

First it is ridiculed,

then it is violently opposed,

finally is accepted as self-evident.

— Arthur Schopenhauer

Homework also includes identifying stakeholders, that is, individuals, groups, and public, private, and other entities affected by the current and/ or the proposed system. Try to anticipate the perceived and actual costs and benefits for each stakeholder and be prepared to acknowledge them. Confirm that the overall "benefits" exceed the overall "costs." This determination typically defies quantification and is likely to require considerable vision and intuition.

Effecting the Change

We "now have our ducks in a row." Our homework is completed, realizing that we may have to occasionally return to the drawing board for refinements. We are ready to advocate a major change within our hospital, company, academic institution, professional society or community group. How should we proceed? Does a sure-fire change model exist? No!

However, one approach that has proven useful is the Awareness-Understanding-Commitment-Action model. It can also be thought of as the Awareness-Head-Heart- Action (AH HA!) approach. The usefulness of this simple model lies in its focus on helping to understand human behavior in a change environment and using that understanding to develop a strategy and tactics to effect change.

- ☐ *Awareness.* Begin by making stakeholders generally **aware** of a possible major change. Go slow and expect widespread disinterest, suspicion, criticism, skepticism, and resistance along with some scattered excitement. Explain why the change is needed. Discuss how the contemplated change would, on the balance, benefit the stakeholders. Don't be discouraged. Machiavelli advises that enmity is expected.

~~~~~~~~~~~~~~~~~~~~~~~~~~~~~~~~~~~~~~~

Carry the battle to them.
Don't let them bring it to you.

— Harry S Truman

▢ *Understanding.* Machiavelli also refers to lukewarm support. Look for, during the awareness step, sources of lukewarm support and focus on those individuals and entities. We should do all we can— ask, listen, talk, meet, write, interact—to help the lukewarm few **understand** why we need the proposed dramatic change and how it will benefit stakeholders. Listen carefully, eliminate semantic hurdles, and refine the proposed change in response to thoughtful concerns and suggestions.

▢ *Commitment.* Have confidence that some lukewarm supporters will become red hot. They will become mentally and emotionally in-volved. Their "heads" and "hearts" will be engaged as they leave wary awareness behind and move through understanding and into commitment. Some will be willing to **commit** their reputations, energy, and creativity by becoming advocates. Urge them to help others understand why the proposed change is needed and how it will benefit stakeholders. This education and interaction effort will start a desirable domino effect in which the commitment of a few expands into the commitment of many. Numerous "heads" and "hearts" will now be on board.

▢ *Action.* Now ask the ever-expanding committed individuals and organizations to go further. Encourage each to **act**, to take at least one step or perform at least one implementation task. Ask each commit-ted individual and organization to place one building block in what is now becoming the foundation of the change superstructure. Step back and quietly and thankfully watch that superstructure rise as more and more stakeholders become aware, achieve understanding, commit and act.

~~~~~~~~~~~~~~~~~~~~~~~~~~~~~

Never doubt that a small group of committed people
can change the world.
It is the only thing that ever has.

— Margaret Mead

While a sharp distinction exists between awareness and understanding and also between understanding and commitment, the differentiation between commitment and action may not be as apparent. The commitment and action steps may appear similar, if not the same. In the absence of action, we may doubt one's commitment.

In response to this concern, there are at least two ways in which bona fide commitment could exist without action. First, while the person may be committed to the change, including the need for it and the benefit of it, he or she may not be familiar enough with the change leaders and their strategies and tactics to be able to identify appropriate acts or tasks. Other individuals may be somewhat introverted (the majority of pharmacists are) and, therefore, somewhat reluctant to step forward and volunteer their services. Learn to recognize these two types of individuals, invite them to act and provide them a task to act on. Offer and then provide support. Be confident that essentially all committed individuals will act if invited to do so and asked to contribute in specific ways.

Widespread Applicability

The four-step process' effectiveness is essentially independent of type of organization within which it is applied. The Awareness-Understanding-Commitment-Action approach will work in the business community, hospitals, academia, professional societies and the non-profit sector. The AH HA! model has broad applicability because it is not highly specific and because it recognizes fundamental human behavior, especially the need to engage head and heart.

Destiny is not a matter of chance,
It is a matter of choice.

— William Jennings Bryan

Suggestions for Applying Ideas

Use the following rules of change to guide your next change effort[2]:

- People can change, but you can't change them. They can change themselves.
- You can only change you.
- When you change, those you interact with have a new experience, increasing the possibility of change for them. Mahatma Gandhi said "be the change you want to see in the world."
- If you don't change, the power to change belongs to others.
- People experience change differently; for some it is exciting. For others, it hurts.
- Organizations, systems, and individuals typically resist change. Lack of change and/or flexibility leads to extinction.
- Identify what will not change, define what will and acknowledge loss.
- Do what you did and you will get what you got.
- Change tends to create conflict, sometimes intense conflict. Poorly managed change creates unnecessary conflict.

Growth demands a temporary surrender of security.

— Gail Sheehy

Because dramatic change is typically proposed to respond to an ominous threat or to seize an unusual opportunity, respond to strong opponents to your proposed change in one of the following ways

◻ Do you agree we are threatened? If so, what change do you propose to meet the threat?

◻ Do you agree we have encountered an opportunity? Is so, how do you propose we seize it or what equivalent or better opportunity do you envision and how do you propose that we pursue it?

◻ The point of the preceding two suggestions: If there is agreement on a threat or opportunity, being against a proposed change to meet the threat or seize the opportunity is not enough. Having an alternative approach is expected.

A jackass can kick down a barn,
but it takes a craftsman to build one.

— Sam Rayburn

Recognize that this lesson addresses ways to effect dramatic change, not continual assessment and improvement

◻ Organizational continual assessment and improvement efforts have many other names including continuous quality improvement and total quality management.

◻ Both types of change are essential in the lives of individuals and organizations. Thriving individuals and organizations, contrasted with those that are just surviving or worse, are adept at effecting both dramatic change when warranted and gradual change through continual assessment and improvement.

◻ Dramatic change requires an intense effort over a short period of time.

◻ The kind of change resulting from assessment and improvement requires a high degree of self and organizational discipline on an ongoing basis. However, because assessment and improvement are highly dependent on individuals, any one of us can begin right now.

How wonderful it is

that nobody need wait a single moment

before starting to improve the world.

— Anne Frank

Read the following related lessons

◻ Lesson 7, "Courage: Real and Counterfeit"

◻ Lesson 8, "Go Out On A Limb"

◻ Lesson 11, "Afraid of Dying, Or Not Having Lived?"

◻ Lesson 44, "Looking Ahead: Can You Spare a Paradigm?"

Study one or more of the following sources cited in this lesson

1. Bergin TG. *Niccolo Machiavelli: The Prince.* Arlington Heights, IL: Crofts Classics; 1947

2. Ganz J. Master the keys to leadership, unlock opportunities. *Engineering Times.* October 2001: 6.

Refer to the following supplemental source

◻ Kriegel R, Brandt D. *Sacred Cows Make the Best Burgers: Paradigm-Busting Strategies for Developing Change-Ready People and Organizations.* New York: Warner Books; 1996.

Visit one or more of these websites

◻ "Emerald for Managers" (http://managers.emeraldinsight.com/index.html) is a website offered by a British firm. Included is a change management page which offers free change-related articles.

◻ "Organisational Change" (http://organisationalchange.co.uk/) is the website of a British firm offering change services such as change management training, organizational change consulting, and TQM training. Articles about change are provided free.

~~~~~~

In a time of drastic change,
it is the learners who inherit the future.
The learned usually find themselves equipped
to live in a world that no longer exists.

— Eric Hoffer

Giving to Our Profession and Our Community

IIIIIIIIIIIIIIIIIIIIIIIIIIIIIIIIIIIIIIIIIIIIIIIIIIIIIIIIIIIIIIIIIIIIIIIIIIIIIIIIII

> *To strive continually for*
> *commitment and involvement*
> *is essential in our pursuit of*
> *excellence.*
>
> — Joseph A. Oddis

Our Profession

Active, as opposed to passive, involvement in professional organizations is one way to continuously increase the value of one's personal professional equity. The process of giving something tangible back to the pharmacy profession helps hone management and leadership ability. Two other effective mechanisms for enhancing personal professional equity are varied and challenging work assignments and continuing education. However, the first half of this lesson focuses on meaningful involvement in professional organizations.

Besides the somewhat selfish concern of maintaining personal professional assets, many of us realize we derive a satisfying and prosperous living from our professions and, accordingly, ought to give something back to them. As practicing pharmacists, we use the work of many predecessor professionals, many of whom produced the books, papers, conference proceedings, manuals of practice, and other valuable contributions for which they received little or no monetary compensation.

As an indication of the contribution of others to the profession and our corresponding obligation to do our share, examine your library or the personal library of another successful pharmacist. Note the relatively large number of materials that were clearly produced, usually in the context of professional organizations, by largely volunteer labor.

I hold every man a debtor to this profession;

from that which man has a course to seek countenance and profit,

so ought they of duty to endeavor themselves,

by way of amends,

to be a help and ornament there unto.

— Francis Bacon

The call to be actively involved in professional organizations goes beyond the benefit of maintaining our currency and the need to meet our obligations. Such participation provides an opportunity to enjoy and benefit from the company of leaders. The healthcare professions and their various subdivisions are like local congregations, mosques or synagogues—many members, very few doers. The doers are usually committed, creative, ambitious, and accomplished people. All of us, but especially the younger professionals, can learn much from associating with leaders. The "ticket" to that club is a commitment to being actively, as opposed to passively, involved in the work of professional organizations.

Once a commitment is made, we face the challenge of identifying the appropriate one or perhaps several professional organizations that we wish to join. Upon becoming a member of such an organization, select one or more types of activities for your involvement and contribution. Besides attending meetings, consider presenting and publishing papers, serving on and chairing committees, helping to arrange and run meetings and conferences and serving as an officer.

By investing our time and talent in one or more professional organizations, we will realize a significant return on our investment in terms of knowledge gained; satisfaction of contribution, that is, giving something back; and association with leaders of our profession.

Our Community

Volunteer efforts, usually quietly and reliably offered, enable many neighborhood, religious, and community organizations to achieve their objectives. How about offering our hard-earned management and leadership skills to assist these organizations?

Many of us know how to make things happen with people in our work environment. We have led and managed teams, departments, offices, projects and programs. Our experience typically includes various forms of spoken and written communication, often sharpened in the challenging and contentious public arena. We have acquired knowledge, skills and attitudes that are directly applicable to and highly valued outside of the workplace. We are well suited for volunteer efforts by virtue of traits such as our orientation toward action, our ability to comprehend the entire system and our knowledge of infrastructure and the environment.

Numerous and varied opportunities exist within our neighborhood-religious-community setting to contribute our time and apply our management talents. Examples are participating in the American Heart Association Heartwalk fund-raiser, serving on an appointed community committee or board, assisting with church or synagogue fund drives, coaching Special Olympics athletes, and running for elective office.

Hospital pharmacists ... should seek increased representation and active participation.

— Herbert L. Flack

Some pharmacists lament, Rodney Dangerfield style, that "we get no respect." Certainly more meaningful visibility in the community by pharmacists would contribute to earning more respect. In a more positive vein, by actively participating in neighborhood, religious, and community groups, we can exert influence and make good things happen. As noted by author Richard Weingardt, "the world is run by those who show up."

Let's share our hard-earned management and leadership knowledge, skills and attitudes to improve our neighborhoods, religious organizations, and our communities. As stated by former British Prime Minister Winston Churchill, "We make a living by what we get, we make a life by what we give."

Suggestions for Applying Ideas

Build a personal development laboratory

Participate in professional and community organizations as way to experiment with your management and leadership strategies and tactics.

- ▢ This is win-win.
- ▢ By stepping in managing and leading roles in volunteer organizations, you incur less economic and professional risk than if you do in your employer's organization.
- ▢ Even if the results are less than you hoped for, the volunteer professional or community organization is likely to benefit from your efforts.

Read the following related lessons

- ▢ Lesson 2, "Roles – Then Goals"
- ▢ Lesson 8, "Go Out on a Limb"
- ▢ Lesson 40, "Eagles and Turkeys"

Refer to the following supplemental source

- Wollenburg KG. Leadership with conscience, compassion, and commitment. *American Journal of Health-System Pharmacy.* 2004;61:1785–1791.

A man there was,
and they called him mad;
the more he gave,
the more he had.

— John Bunyan

Looking Ahead: Can You Spare a Paradigm?

Sacred cows make the best burgers.

— Robert Kriegel and David Brandt

We should, as individuals and as organizations, be preparing ourselves for the way our profession will be practiced, not the way it is or was practiced. Looking well into the early 21st century, the work force will be increasingly heterogeneous with balanced participation by men and women at all levels and with greater participation by ethnic minorities, and seniors. Future pharmacists and other healthcare professionals will increasingly serve patients with new diagnostic and therapeutic modalities. Finally, the logistics of work will change with movement toward computerized prescribing and automated dispensing, a more varied education-work-retirement pattern, shorter tenure within organizations, and for the proactive, attainment of career security. However, our basic mission will not change; we will continue to focus on meeting society's pharmaceutical care needs.

Anticipating the future is, at best, very difficult. An important quality is being able to "take off the blinders" which naturally leads to the topic of paradigms. Speaker and author Stephen Covey[1] defines a paradigm as "The way we 'see' the world—not in terms of our visual sense of sight, but in terms of perceiving, understanding, and interpreting." According to futur-ist Joel Barker a paradigm is "a set of rules and regulations that... defines boundaries and tells you what to do to be successful within those bound-aries."[2] Psychologists Robert Kriegel and David Brandt suggest that a paradigm is like the sandbox you played in as a child—it was your world.[3]

Paradigms abound; they are all around us, as seen from the following examples:

- ▫ Pharmacist's role in computer entry of medication orders
- ▫ Residency training for advance clinical roles
- ▫ Pharmacokinetic monitoring of medication with a narrow therapeu-tic index
- ▫ Bar code use in medication distribution

Paradigms are very useful, given the complexity of society. They almost always allow for more than one "right" answer. For example, there are many ways to interpret paradigms such as the pharmacist's clinical role and preferred technology for medication distribution.

What we believe our profession
to be determines what it is.

— Wendell T. Hill, Jr.

On the negative side, Joel Barker claims that paradigms tend to reverse the "seeing and believing" process. Intelligent, thoughtful people like to think that they are rational, that they "believe because they see." However, because of paradigms, people often "see because they believe." Consider, for example, some beliefs you hold and have held for a long time and highly value. Are you not likely to find many examples of situations which tend to support your belief and might you not actually be looking for them? And might you be "seeing because you believe" rather than "believing because you see?" As noted by marketing and communications consultant

H. Jackson Brown, Jr., "We do not see things as they are. We see things as we are."

Unfortunately, if paradigms are too strongly held, and they often are, the holders risk incurring paradigm paralysis. Paradigm pliancy is a much better strategy, according to Barker, especially in turbulent times. Pliancy is a quality or state of yielding or changing. Fortunately, at least a handful of people in any organization can change their paradigms. Even for them, however, paradigm pliancy is at best difficult.

You can never plan the future
by the past.

— Edmund Burke

As suggested by the abacus–slide rule–electronic calculator–digital computer progression, paradigms do shift. Many examples can be found within clinical professions and throughout society at large. Paradigms vanish and new ones replace them.

What does the future hold? The most successful individuals and organizations avoid paradigm paralysis—they will practice paradigm pliancy. They will create new paradigms and build bridges to them or at least recognize new paradigms when they are coming down the pike and see the business and professional opportunities within them. Thriving individuals and organizations practice paradigm pliancy. In contrast, paradigm paralysis characterizes individuals and organizations satisfied with surviving or in the process of dying. What paradigms will you contribute to your clinical field or, what paradigms created by others will you enthusiastically embrace and advance?

When all is said and done, there are only two futures for individuals and organizations. The first is the future we create for ourselves. The second is the future others create for us. If we, as individuals or organizations don't choose the first, others will impose the second.

Suggestions for Applying Ideas

Identify possible paradigms shifts by comparing situations that existed several decades ago in the U.S. to those that exist today

- Inter-high school and college sports were essentially exclusively for males.[2]

- The slide rule was the personal computer—a digital computer with its peripherals typically filled an entire room. Mr. Ken Olsen, former President of Digital Electronic Corporation, a computer manufacturer, said "There is no reason for any individual to have a computer in their home."[4]

- There was a strong feeling that nuclear power would soon solve most energy problems throughout the U.S. and that many nuclear power plants would be built in successive decades.[2]

- Mail routinely took days to be delivered.

- The worldwide conflicts between democracy and communism and capitalism and socialism would continue forever.

- Most pharmaceutical representatives were pharmacists.

All of the preceding paradigms have vanished having been replaced by new paradigms.

Each of us needs to shift our paradigm or it will be shifted for us.

— Marianne Ivey

Consider some of the paradigm shifts of the last few decades, with emphasis on the "shifters," "outsiders," and "odd balls" responsible for them.

- Fred Smith founded Federal Express[2,4] so that mail, in the U.S. at least, could be routinely delivered overnight. As a Yale University student, Smith wrote a paper proposing overnight mail delivery in the U.S. using trucks and airplanes operating within a hub and spoke system. According to the professor who gave Mr. Smith a "C" on the paper, the idea was interesting, but would never work.

☐ High jumper Dick Fosbury was ridiculed for leading with his head at a time when all others jumped feet first. However, the ridiculed "Fosbury flop" enabled Fosbury to win the high-jump gold medal in 1968 at Mexico City. Leading with the head is now the standard for world-class high jumpers.[3]

☐ W. Edwards Deming's advice on what is now called total quality management was ignored by American businesses. Under the auspices of the U.S. government, he assisted the Japanese after World War II who, in a matter of a few decades, set the world standard for manufactured products.[2]

Do not follow where the path may lead.
Go instead where there is no path and leave a trail.

— Anonymous

Examine, at the most fundamental level, the assumptions, approaches, techniques, and tools you use in your professional work and, perhaps, beyond

The "you" in this advice applies to individuals and organizations. What are you doing simply because you have "always" done it? Driven by your vision, and consistent with your mission and core values, what could and should be cast out and replaced? What might you try to do that you are not doing? Some ideas for individuals and/or organizations are as follows:

☐ Stop thinking first of why something can't be done; think instead of ways to do it.

☐ Revisit your organization's "bigger is better" strategy. Might fewer employees filling crucial or core clinical, managing and leading roles be more productive, more profitable, less stressful, more enjoyable and otherwise better? This assumes they would be supported by technology and pharmacy technicians.

- Assume full responsibility for the quality and efficiency of medication use.

- Assure that a pharmacist speaks with every patient about his or her medications.

- Establish collaborative practice agreements to expand the pharmacist's role in medication management.

The overall idea is to occasionally examine, in a fresh and critical manner, the basics of what we are doing. This goes beyond continuous improvement, as important as that is. The goal is to find those aspects of our work life and beyond, that could and maybe should be radically changed for our benefit and the benefit of our employers, our customers and others within our circle of influence.

Refer to the following related lessons

- Lesson 8, "Go Out On A Limb"
- Lesson 11, "Afraid of Dying, Or Having Not Lived?"
- Lesson 25, "We Don't Make Whitewalls: Work Smarter, Not Harder"
- Lesson 42, "AH HA! A Process for Effecting Change"

Study one or more of the following sources cited in this lesson

1. Covey S. *The 7 Habits of Highly Effective People.* New York, NY: Simon & Schuster; 1990: 23.

2. Barker JA. *Discovering the Future: The Business of Paradigms.* St. Paul, MN: IL Press; 1989.

3. Kriegel R, Brandt D. *Sacred Cows Make the Best Burgers.* New York: Warner Books; 1996: 56.

4. Cypert SA. *The Success Breakthrough.* New York: Avon Books; 1993: 201–202.

Refer to the following supplemental source

◻ Ivey MF. Harvey A. K. Whitney lecture. Shifting pharmacy's paradigm *American Journal of Health-System Pharmacy.* 50:1869–1874.

*I believe that pharmacy will be at health care's
center stage in the next century,
and that there will be a standing ovation
and rave reviews.*

— William A. Gouveia

Appendix

Sources of Quotations
‖‖

Numbers refer to the lesson that contains a quotation by the individual listed. Unless otherwise noted, individuals are from the United States.

A

Konrad ADENAUER, Chancellor of the Federal Republic of Germany, 11

AESOP, Greek slave who authored fables, 7

Thomas Bailey ALDRICH, father of the American novel, 20

James ALLEN, English writer, 26

Mary Ann ALLISON, business author, 38

Neil ARMSTRONG, astronaut, 15

Marcus AURELIUS, Roman philosopher-emperor, 26

B

Francis BACON, English philosopher and statesman, 20, 43

Byrd BAGGETT, salesman, 6

Homa BAHRAMI, educator, speaker, author, 10

C

Index